Patrick Holford is a leading spokesman on nutrition in the media and is the author of over 30 books, including *The Optimum Nutrition Bible*. In 1984 he founded the Institute for Optimum Nutrition (ION), an independent educational trust for the furtherance of education and research in nutrition. He is chief executive of the Food for the Brain Foundation and an honorary fellow of the British Association for Applied Nutrition and Nutritional Therapy.

Natalie Savona is a writer, television presenter and the author of various other books, including *Wonderfoods* and *The Kitchen Shrink*. A graduate of the Institute for Optimum Nutrition (ION) and Cambridge University, Natalie has now turned her research to how our food choices reflect our psychological and cultural influences.

Other books by Patrick Holford

Patrick Holford has written about a wide variety of health issues. To make it easier to identify the subjects that may interest you, his key titles have been categorised into the following general subject areas:

Essentials

The Optimum Nutrition Bible
Optimum Nutrition Made Easy (with Susannah Lawson)
The Optimum Nutrition Cookbook (with Judy Ridgway)
Optimum Nutrition Before, During and After Pregnancy (with Susannah Lawson)

Weight

The Low-GL Diet Bible
The Low-GL Diet Made Easy
The Low-GL Diet Cookbook (with Fiona McDonald Joyce)
Food GLorious Food (with Fiona McDonald Joyce)

Mind

The Feel Good Factor
Optimum Nutrition for the Mind
The Alzheimer's Prevention Plan (with Shane Heaton and Deborah Colson)
Smart Foods for Smart Kids (with Fiona McDonald Joyce)
Optimum Nutrition for Your Child (with Deborah Colson)

Body

Say No to Diabetes
How to Quit Without Feeling S★★t (with David Miller and Dr James Braly)
Food is Better Medicine Than Drugs (with Jerome Burne)
The Holford 9-Day Liver Detox (with Fiona McDonald Joyce)
Say No to Arthritis
Say No to Cancer
Say No to Heart Disease
Beat Stress and Fatigue
Boost Your Immune System (with Jennifer Meek)
Improve Your Digestion

patrick
HOLFORD
& Natalie Savona

SOLVE YOUR
SKIN
PROBLEMS

piatkus

PIATKUS

First published in Great Britain in 2001 by Piatkus Books
Reprinted 2005, 2006, 2007 (twice), 2009, 2010, 2011, 2013, 2014

A CIP catalogue record for this book
is available from the British Library.

ISBN 978-0-7499-2185-9

Typeset in Bembo by Phoenix Photosetting, Chatham, Kent
Printed and bound by CPI Group (UK) Ltd, Croydon, CR0 4YY

Papers used by Piatkus are from well-managed forests
and other responsible sources.

MIX
Paper from
responsible sources
FSC® C104740

Piatkus
An imprint of
Little, Brown Book Group
100 Victoria Embankment
London EC4Y 0DY

An Hachette UK Company
www.hachette.co.uk

www.piatkus.co.uk

CONTENTS

Acknowledgements   vii
Guide to Abbreviations and Measures   viii
References and Further Sources of Information   viii
How to Use this Book   ix

PART 1   UNDERSTANDING YOUR SKIN

1   What is Your Skin?   3
2   Strength and Suppleness   11
3   Skin Damage – Understanding Oxidation   14
4   Sun – Your Skin's Enemy   19
5   Teens and Menopause – the Critical Years   25
6   Nail Signals   31

PART 2   BEAUTY IS MORE THAN SKIN-DEEP

7   Digestion – the Key to Health   35
8   Detox for Clear Skin   43
9   Skin Saviours – Understanding Antioxidants   50
10   Essential Skin Oils   60

PART 3 SKIN SOLUTIONS

11 Acne   69
12 Acne Rosacea   77
13 Skin Healing   82
14 Skin Cancer   86
15 Psoriasis   90
16 Eczema and Dermatitis   98
17 Cellulite   106
18 Rashes and Hives   113
19 Cold Sores   121
20 Fungal Infections   125
21 Other Skin Conditions   128

PART 4 ACTIVE SKIN REJUVENATION

22 Eat Yourself Beautiful   137
23 Water – Nature's Moisturiser   142
24 Detoxifying Your Skin   145
25 Low-reaction Diets   151
26 Supplements for Clear Skin   155
27 External Skincare   158

References   166
Recommended Reading   171
Useful Addresses   173
Index   177

ACKNOWLEDGEMENTS

I would like to thank Natalie for being a co-author from heaven, and we are both indebted to the team at Piatkus, including Rachel Winning, Katie Andrews and Kelly Davis, our editor.

Patrick Holford

My deepest thanks go to Isabelle Legeron for her unwavering support while I was working on this book. Also, to Patrick for asking me to write with him in the first place; Sally Penford at the International Dermal Institute for sharing her vast expertise; and Valerie Holmes for providing invaluable information on antioxidants.

Natalie Savona

Guide to abbreviations and measures

1 gram (g) = 1000 milligrams (mg) = 1,000,000 micrograms (mcg or μg). Most vitamins are measured in milligrams or micrograms. Vitamins A, D and E are also measured in International Units (iu), a measurement designed to standardise the different forms of these vitamins which have different potencies.

1mcg of retinol (mcg RE) = 3.3iu of vitamin A (RE = Retinol Equivalents)

1mcg RE of beta-carotene = 6mcg of beta-carotene

100iu of vitamin D = 2.5mcg

100iu of vitamin E = 67mg

1 pound (lb) = 16 ounces (oz)

2.2lb = 1 kilogram (kg)

1 pint = 0.6 litres

1.76 pints = 1 litre

2 teaspoons (tsp) = 1 dessertspoon (dsp)

1.5 dessertspoons = 1 tablespoon (tbsp)

References and further sources of information

Hundreds of references from respected scientific literature have been used in writing this book. Details of specific studies referred to are listed on pages 167–71. Other supporting research for statements made is available from the Lamberts Library at the Institute for Optimum Nutrition (ION), see page 175, whose members are free to visit and study there. ION also offers information services, including literature and library search facilities, for readers who would like to access scientific literature on specific subjects. On pages 172–3 you will find a list of books to read to follow up information in this book.

How To Use This Book

This book is about having fantastic-looking skin by keeping it young and healthy – from the inside out.

Part 1 takes an in-depth look at what your skin really is (how it's made and how it works), then Part 2 explores some vital (but often forgotten) factors linked to nutrition which are fundamental to good skin. Part 3 gives no-nonsense information on a wide range of specific skin conditions, explaining their underlying causes and giving practical suggestions for their treatment. Finally, Part 4 gives general, easy-to-follow recommendations for getting your skin looking good and keeping it that way.

PART 1

UNDERSTANDING YOUR SKIN

CHAPTER 1

....

WHAT IS YOUR SKIN?

Your skin may just feel like a case for your body, with some hair here, a few bumps and creases there; a mere shield that protects you from the world outside. But it's more than just the stuff that keeps your insides in – it's actually a remarkably complex organ which reflects your total health. So, by keeping your skin looking great, you are also keeping your insides in good order and slowing down the ageing process. In order to keep your skin glowing, smooth and healthy, it helps to have some idea of how it works and all the roles it plays in your body.

By learning what goes on in your skin, you will find it easier to understand how much its condition is influenced by what you eat and drink, as well as by other factors such as your environment and the cosmetics you use. Whether you have spots or a more serious condition, or you just want to maintain an already youthful complexion, this book explains how to keep your skin super-healthy and young-looking, and to recognise why things may be going wrong and what to do about it.

Your skin is, after all, the largest organ in your body: in an adult it weighs around 5 kg (11 lb), which is as much as a dog, and has a surface area of 2 square metres (22 square feet), about the size of a double bed. No other organ is so exposed to damage or disease from the outside – from injury, sunlight, smoking, environmental pollution and germs. At the same time, your skin also reflects internal conditions and emotions, for example when it blushes or sweats.

Some skin disorders (such as warts) are confined just to the skin, while others – indeed most of them – reflect what is going on inside. For instance, cold sores and chicken pox show that your immune system is fighting off an internal infection, a rash may be the result of an allergic reaction to a food you have eaten, and a yellowish skin tone may indicate that there is a problem with your liver. Clearly, the condition of your skin depends on a number of factors including your age, genes, hygiene, circulation, immune system, environment, psychological state and, of course, what you eat.

WHAT DOES YOUR SKIN DO?

Apart from providing a container for the rest of your body, your skin is involved – through the nerves – in sensing touch, temperature changes and other sensations such as itching and pain. It also regulates your body temperature by dilating blood vessels near its surface when your brain signals it to cool down, or by contracting the blood vessels when it needs to retain heat. In addition, your skin both absorbs and eliminates various oils and liquids, protects you from infection and produces vitamin D. This diversity of roles gives some insight into the skin's complex nature. It also shows how intricately the way your skin works and looks is linked to what is going on internally. In this sense your skin is a barometer of your inner environment.

This is why effective skincare, which aims to keep skin looking good and free from any problems, cannot merely come from the outside. The condition of our skin is very important to our self-image – it is, after all, the part of us that other people see – as shown by the amount of time and money some people spend on trying to keep it looking youthful. Most of this money is, however, spent on products which are applied externally and, although there is definitely a role for beauty and medical creams, it is crucial to nourish the skin from the inside too. To see why this is so important, it is helpful to understand a little about the structure of skin and the way it works.

THE STRUCTURE OF THE SKIN

The epidermis

The layer of tissue that we call skin can broadly be divided into two layers – the dermis ('skin' in Latin) and the epidermis ('outside skin'). Underneath the dermis is a layer of fat cells called the subcutaneous fat, which adds to the skin's protective cushion.

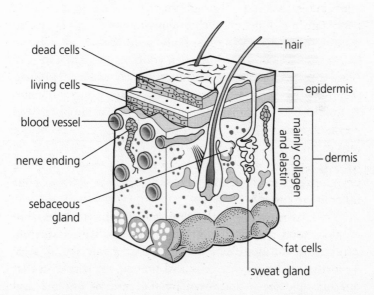

Figure 1 – The structure of the skin (cross-section)

The epidermis has four layers (see Figure 1). The outer-most of these – the stratum corneum or 'horny layer' – is made up of stacked, flat cells that are more or less dead. They consist mainly of a strong protein called keratin, produced by cells called keratinocytes, and different types of lipids (oils). Their protein and fat content is very important in helping the epidermis to hold in moisture and to allow substances to pass out of the body. The cells are thin and tough; they gradually fall off or are rubbed off as we go about our daily lives, making way for others to take their place. Amazingly, this layer of cells which is our interface with the outside world, which helps control what passes in and out of our skin, is thinner than a human hair.

The cells in the stratum corneum are originally formed in the basal layer and gradually work their way up to the surface, changing their structure and content as they do. The rate at which the cells progress from the basal layer into the outer-most part of the skin varies from person to person, but the epidermis is completely renewed in anything from six to ten weeks. In some people this process is disrupted and happens far too quickly and they develop psoriasis (see Chapter 15). The epidermis also contains cells which produce melanin (one of the substances that is responsible for colouring the skin), as well as cells which play a part in the skin's immune reaction.

The dermis

The dermis actually makes up the vast majority of the skin. In addition to living cells, the outer layer of the dermis contains blood vessels, connective tissue, lymph vessels and some elastin and collagen fibres (more on these later). The layer beneath this has fewer cells and vessels but much greater amounts of collagen and elastin. The dermis also contains hair follicles, sebaceous glands and sweat glands which open out as pores on the skin's surface, as well as nerves that are sensitive to pressure and pain.

Sebaceous glands

Sebaceous glands are sack-like structures that open into hair follicles (or directly on to the skin in some places); they are found all over the body except on the palms, soles and tops of the feet. The size of the glands varies between different body parts. For example, they are bigger on the face and chest but smaller on the arms and legs.

These glands produce sebum, an oily substance which helps stop hair drying out and becoming brittle. It also keeps the skin oily (to prevent too much evaporation of water), soft and free of some bacteria (although it can feed others). One of the reasons that spots and acne are more common amongst teenagers is that sebum secretion is partly controlled by hormones, and an excess can block pores which may then become infected (see Chapter 11). Blackheads are the result of a build-up in pores of sebum combined with melanin.

Skin colour

If you stop and look around you at people's skin colours, you'll notice how many different hues there are. The colours in any biological matter – and that includes our skin – depend on the complex molecules of which it is made. Skin derives its colour largely from three pigments – melanin, carotene and haemoglobin.

Melanin This is the main determinant of colour – giving anything from a pale yellow to black skin – and is produced by cells called melanocytes. These are most plentiful in the mucous membranes, penis, nipples, the area around the nipples, face, limbs and parts of the eye. The number of melanocytes is more or less the same in all races – it's the amount of melanin the cells produce for distribution to the keratinocytes that determines how dark the skin is. It works by enveloping the cells' DNA, and absorbing harmful ultra-violet light (see Chapter 4).

Carotene This is the yellowy-orange pigment that gives egg yolks, carrots and other vegetables their colour. It is transformed in the body into vitamin A, which is needed for vision.

Haemoglobin The red colour in skin is due to the haemo-globin in the capillaries near the surface. Haemoglobin is the molecule that carries oxygen in blood. If the blood is not picking up enough oxygen from the lungs for any reason, the skin will look slightly blueish.

Sweat glands

Whether we like it or not, sweating is an important, normal bodily process. Its main function is to prevent the body from getting too hot and it also helps us eliminate some waste products. There are as many as four million sweat glands spread all over the body, most densely in the palms of the hands and the soles of the feet. In response to overheating, a complex nervous mechanism triggers the secretion of water and several other substances up through the sweat glands which each open out into a pore on the skin's surface.

Lymph vessels

The lymphatic system (Figure 2) is made up of vessels that run all over the body. Indeed, it has been said that if you were to remove absolutely every part of someone except their lymph vessels, you would still be able to recognise them. Through these vessels flows lymph fluid which carries out various func-tions, including carrying waste products from your cells,

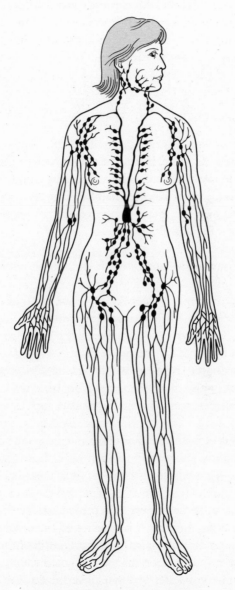

Figure 2 – The lymphatic system

transporting substances between cells and draining the excess fluid that gathers between the body's cells. While doing this, the lymph fluid also filters foreign organisms and other matter, and traps them in the lymph nodes where they are attacked – which is why you get 'swollen glands' if you are unwell. In addition, the lymphatic system transports fats and fat-soluble vitamins (A, D, E and K) which are absorbed through the gut.

Unlike the blood system, the lymph does not have a pump in the form of the heart. Instead, the lymph moves around the body with the help of the body movements themselves – one good reason for exercising regularly. As the tissues surrounding the lymph move, they compress and release the vessels, pushing the fluid along.

If the body has a good water supply, by taking in plenty of pure water and adequate protein, the lymph system works very efficiently. If, however, water intake is low, fat intake is excessive (common in developed countries) and protein intake is inadequate (rare in developed countries), lymph flow is impaired, which means that the body's cleansing system is not on top form. So, in addition to pressure – from injury, standing for long periods, or whatever – diet plays an important role in lymph function, which in turn will affect the body's clearing of waste and its water balance.

Clearly, your skin is not just a container for your body – it is very much a living organ in its own right. It is only its location that gives it a whole different set of factors to deal with in keeping healthy. There is also the fact that the body automatically prioritises those organs that are essential to life, such as the heart and brain (giving precedence to them in the supply of blood, water and nutrients, and leaving the skin until last). This is why it is so important for the health of your skin to make sure that your diet includes plentiful supplies of all the vital nutrients.

CHAPTER 2

STRENGTH AND SUPPLENESS

The remarkable strength of your skin and its ability to stretch (and to return to its original shape after being stretched) are due to two components of the dermis: collagen and elastin. The skin stretches, for example, in pregnancy, in obese people, as a result of some injuries, and even in stretching and flexing your elbow. Red stretch marks (or striae) can appear when stretching is extreme enough to tear the dermis, although afterwards only silvery streaks remain as a sign of the damage.

COLLAGEN

The most abundant tissue in the body is connective tissue, which, as its name suggests, binds, supports and strengthens other tissues. Collagen is the name given to one type of connective tissue. It forms about three-quarters of the skin's dry weight, so keeping it healthy is vital to having good skin. The word comes from the Greek *kolla* which means 'glue'. For centuries glue was made from the hide of animals – in the same way collagen effectively 'holds us together'. It is a tough, rigid substance made up of bundled fibres of protein which do not stretch very much. Its rigidity and ability to respond to physical stresses lessen with age and exposure to sunlight (for more on the sun's effects on skin, see Chapter 4). Vitamin C is essential for the formation of the key protein in collagen – hydroxyproline. This is why some of the symptoms of scurvy (caused by vitamin C deficiency) include cracked skin, bleeding gums and poor wound healing. Without vitamin C the skin cannot maintain its structure.

ELASTIN

In contrast to collagen, elastin – the other major structural protein in skin – has a 'spring' to it. It too provides the skin with strength but, as its name suggests, elastin is what gives skin its resilience; it allows skin (and other tissues such as the lungs and blood vessel walls) to expand and spring back to its normal size. The fibres that make up elastin can be stretched to one-and-a-half times their relaxed length without breaking. To see this for yourself, just pull your ear lobe down and see how much its surface area expands.

It is believed to be changes in the structure of elastin which result in wrinkles[1] although, structurally speaking, little difference has been found in the actual cells of wrinkly skin and smooth skin.[2] What actually causes this damage appears to be oxidation, which is explained fully in Chapter 3. So wrinkles are actually caused by a combination of factors: damage to cells through oxidation and the body's natural ageing process which gradually reduces its ability to retain its structure.

Collagen and elastin are contained in a fluid which is made up of several substances including water, and this is one reason why a good water intake is so important for maintaining healthy, supple skin.

KEEPING YOUR SKIN STRONG AND SUPPLE

As we have seen, the health of your skin (and all parts of your body) depends significantly on what you take in. For instance, you need adequate vitamin C for collagen formation, you need sufficient water to keep the cells of your skin hydrated, and you need adequate nutrients to maintain the structure of your skin. Next, though, we need to look at another major factor which affects skin condition – both internally and externally – oxidation damage.

CHAPTER 3

....

SKIN DAMAGE – UNDERSTANDING OXIDATION

L eave an apple that has fallen from a tree on the ground in the sun and it will soon shrivel up and go brown. While our skin, unlike the apple, has a constant supply of nourishment from within (assuming we eat and drink well), the effects of the sun and air nevertheless take their toll. As our outermost, protective layer, our skin is constantly exposed to chemicals and environmental factors which influence its health and appearance. These factors include chemicals in the air and from cigarette smoke, chlorine from swimming pools, extreme temperatures and ultraviolet radiation from the sun.

On top of these external factors, various internal bodily processes bring on the signs of ageing too – even people who live in clean environments and don't sunbathe get wrinkles as they age. So what is it that actually damages the skin, turning it from that smooth, taut face we are born with to the lined, wrinkled face most people end up with? Well, the culprit is oxidative damage, caused by free oxidising radicals or oxidants (sometimes known as free radicals) for short.[3] They come from pollution, cigarette smoke, fried and burnt foods, processed cooking oils, sunlight, combustion and, ironically, the body's own burning of oxygen to produce energy. Just as oxygen can damage iron to form rust, so it can damage molecules in our bodies. Oxidants have been linked to the increase in heart disease, cancer, Alzheimer's and many more diseases as well as general ageing.[4] Indeed, people with Down's Syndrome, who age more quickly, have been found to have a defect in the way their bodies deal with oxidants.[5]

HOW DOES OXIDATION OCCUR?

Oxidants are the body's equivalent of nuclear waste which must be decommissioned to remove the danger. We can think of them as the sparks generated by our bodies burning glucose to make energy in our cells, or by pollution. These sparks, or oxidants, cause damage and need to be put out. The spark extinguishers are the 'antioxidants'.

Without going into all the technical details, here's a brief explanation of how they wreak their havoc. First, imagine millions of atoms, in our bodies, and in the chemicals in the environment. Each atom has paired positive and negative charges (electrons) which keep it nicely balanced. An oxidant is, in contrast, unbalanced and highly reactive. It is an atom with one of its charges missing, so it causes chaos by trying to grab one from a nearby atom. As you can imagine, the theft of an electron itself creates another oxidant and so the process continues in a cascade of damage.

Ironically, most of the oxidants in the body are actually toxic forms of one of our most essential elements – oxygen. Think of what happens when iron is exposed to oxygen – it rusts. Likewise, when a piece of apple is left exposed – it goes brown. Similarly, oxygen can cause damage in our bodies.

Oxidants are very destructive overall because they damage fats, proteins, connective tissue and nucleic acids (DNA and RNA). The parts of our bodies which are particularly vulnerable to such attack are the membranes of our cells and the DNA within them. The cell membrane is responsible for controlling what goes in and out of cells – nutrients, water, hormones, toxins, etc – so any damage to this can affect the way the cell works. DNA (deoxyribonucleic acid) is our individual blueprint which exists in each cell. Damage to this interferes with the instructions the cell gives for producing new cells and for making essential substances such as hormones or enzymes.

MINIMISING YOUR EXPOSURE TO OXIDANTS

A recent advertising campaign in the London Underground showed a telling image – an ashtray filled with ash and a large make-up brush, alongside the slogan: 'Clinically proven to give you grottier-looking skin.' It goes on to say, 'There's certainly one product that guarantees fast, effective results when it comes to skin care. Every cigarette contains special active ingredients called "toxins" that constrict blood vessels, starve your skin of oxygen and remove lingering traces of a healthy complexion. In fact, the only thing glowing about your face will be the cigarette end.'

We are all well aware that smoking is bad for us, and oxidation is one of the main reasons why. The process of the tobacco burning involved in smoking is a major source of oxidants in smokers and even in passive smokers. Not only does this affect the lungs and the rest of the body (including the skin) internally but also the skin on the outside. A research study published in 1999 showed that cigarette smoking causes a breakdown in elastin – the substance which gives skin its elasticity – resulting in more wrinkles and discoloration in smokers' skin.[6]

Smoking is particularly bad for the skin for two other main reasons. The first is that it interferes with the blood flow to the capillaries – the tiny blood vessels that take oxygen and nutrients to the skin and carry away carbon dioxide and waste products. This inevitably diminishes the health and function of the skin. A study in Israel showed that smoking interferes with the blood supply to capillaries which feed the skin and extremities.[7] A second reason is that the actual action of drawing on a cigarette may increase the development of lines around the mouth.

Like smoking, air pollution (generated by car exhausts, factory emissions, and so on) promotes oxidation in your skin. Exposure to ozone was shown in a clinical study on mice to cause damage to the skin and its natural oils due to the build-up of oxidants.[8]

What causes oxidation?

- tobacco smoke.

- exhaust fumes.

- industrial pollution.

- burnt, brown or fried food.

- excessive exposure to the sun.

- radiation.

- viruses and bacteria.

- energy production in the body.

- pesticides.

- aromatic hydrocarbons (petroleum-based products).

- alcohol.

As you can see from this list, not all sources of oxidants are avoidable. However, we *can* choose not to smoke or to spend time in smoky environments, to minimise the time we are in traffic, not to exercise near busy roads, to avoid fried or burnt food and to stay out of the sun. The sun is a major, avoidable source of skin damage, which is discussed fully in the next chapter.

UNAVOIDABLE OXIDANTS

Yet, even without being exposed to external factors that cause oxidant damage, our metabolism generates them itself, as toxic byproducts of its own intricate system of energy production. So, if they are so dangerous, why do our bodies manufacture them? Well, some are actually used in other processes – for instance, to help kill harmful organisms and malignant cells, and to help in blood clotting.

The body has some very sophisticated ways of dealing with oxidants – a battery of defence enzymes called, as you proba-bly know, antioxidants. It is therefore generally well equipped to deal with the oxidants it produces itself. Problems only arise – in the form of skin damage or disease, from ageing to cancer – when these internal mechanisms are overburdened, faulty or not given adequate nutrient support.

A great deal of recent medical research has focused on the role of antioxidants in preventing disease and delaying ageing. Chapter 9 explains fully how to maximise your antioxidant potential, and also examines the role of antioxidants in health.

In summary, to reduce damage to your skin through oxidation:

- Avoid or limit your exposure to external oxidative factors, such as those listed on page 17.

- Stop smoking.

- Eat plenty of antioxidant-rich foods (see Chapter 9).

- Take an antioxidant supplement (see Chapter 9).

CHAPTER 4

SUN – YOUR SKIN'S ENEMY

There are various theories on why so many of us are so keen to roast ourselves in the sun at any available opportunity. One is that Coco Chanel set a trend after getting a tan during a visit to St Tropez in the south of France, thus destroying the association of brown skin with lowly peasants who spent their lives working the land. Another is that, during the Prohibition era, those who could afford to, visited off-shore islands to drink, returning home with a suntan and a case full of contraband – making darker skin into a status symbol. Whichever you believe, recent evidence shows that it is only the fools among us who still fall for this and a suntan is merely the body's response to danger.

For many years now, we have been aware of the need to stay out of the sun and use sunscreens. Vanity and fashion, however, dictate otherwise. Most of us 'feel better' when we have a tan – particularly psychologically – and pay good money to spend our annual holiday soaking it up.

THE A, B, C OF ULTRAVIOLET

The sun emits many different types of rays. Luckily the stratosphere and ozone filter out shorter rays. If ozone didn't filter out ultraviolet C, for example, we would not be here, as it destroys DNA. Ultraviolet A and B (two of the longer rays) are of particular concern, although others (such as infrared) are increasingly being implicated in skin damage too.

UVB rays are shorter than UVA, and they are the ones which cause most damage, although both are harmful.[9] UVB rays penetrate the epidermis and are known as the rays which cause burning. They oxidise the fats in the cell membranes, ruining their barrier function. Some UVB rays manage to get further into the epidermis, causing sunburn which is, in effect, oxidative damage (see Chapter 3) to the DNA and other proteins. The redness and inflammation caused by sunburn are a result of the oxidation and the dilation of blood vessels as the skin attempts to protect and repair itself. This goes on long after the initial sun exposure and the cascade of oxidants sets the scene for potentially cancerous cell changes later on.

UVA rays cause oxidative damage to cells and the connective tissue in the dermis, which leads to burning and ageing. Initially believed to be less harmful than UVB, it is now known that UVA rays can penetrate further into the skin, into the dermis, where they damage collagen and elastin. With these two important connective tissues destroyed, it is not difficult to see the link between UVA exposure and ageing. UVA rays are, in a way, more insidious because they get through to the skin even on a cloudy day and through glass, unlike UVB which can only reach the surface of the earth when the sun is high in the sky.

All the different rays aside, the bottom line is that UV light damages our cells on a molecular level: it interferes with their ability to make proteins and reproduce properly, speeds up the replication of damaged cells, harms the collagen and elastin which normally keep our skin strong and elastic, breaks down the important fats in the cell membrane, and ultimately creates a dry, rapidly ageing skin which is even more susceptible to further damage.

These effects have worsened in recent years because the amount of UV light reaching the earth's surface is increasing as the protective ozone layer is being depleted, due to chemical reactions between it and various chemicals (chlorofluorocarbons or CFCs) found in refrigerators and some spray cans. Also, the closer you get to the sun, the more susceptible you are to the effects of UV rays, so it's even more important to protect yourself from the sun when mountain climbing, skiing or visiting high altitudes.

NATURAL DEFENCES

In the face of this onslaught from the sun, our bodies do have remarkable protective mechanisms. The first defence that comes into play, but only if we carefully control our exposure to the sun, is melanin, the pigment produced in the skin. It absorbs light, and, as exposure continues, more melanin is produced by the melanocytes, creating a suntan. People with darker skin have more melanin, so they are more resistant to the harmful effects of the sun, while albinos have no melanin at all, so they burn severely in even the slightest sun exposure. The keratinocytes also play a protective role by moving the protective pigments – melanin and keratin – towards your skin's surface to provide your very own sunscreen.

Shiny, wet skin absorbs more light than dry skin because of the way the rays bend through liquid. This is why putting oil on your skin before sunbathing is likely to increase tanning. Cell membranes in the skin (which are partly composed of oils) are particularly susceptible to damage from UV rays, and it is now accepted that long-term exposure to UV light accelerates the ageing process and the risk of skin cancer.

Unfortunately, melanin is not enough to protect us from the damage caused by the sun. In many people it 'mutinies' and dumps melanin in clusters which show up as freckles. The sun causes permanent damage by oxidising the elastin in skin – the proteins become cross-linked and lose their elasticity. To understand the effect, picture the perished rubber of an old flip-flop which has been lying on a beach exposed to sunlight – instead of being flexible, it is hard and crumbly. The DNA in your cells is also very susceptible to damage. And the havoc caused by damaged DNA is believed to be a major cause of cancer. It also prevents the DNA from sending accurate messages to cells, resulting in changes to the structure of the skin, leaving it less supple, dryer and eventually rather rough and wrinkly. This sort of damage is irreversible.

Another clever defence mechanism the skin employs to protect itself from the sun is altering its thickness. In response to continued attack by UVB (not UVA), the stratum corneum – which, you may remember, largely consists of dead, keratin-filled cells – gets thicker. These dead cells offer protection from the sun by absorbing or reflecting a significant amount of UVB.

Our third line of defence is the body's own antioxidants, such as vitamins A, C and E, and enzymes which 'mop up' some of the oxidant damage caused by the sun. These, however, only have a limited life and are rapidly over-run after just a few minutes in fierce sun. Recent research published by the American Academy of Dermatology showed that sunburn was reduced by taking vitamin C (2000 mg) and vitamin E (1000 iu), both potent antioxidant nutrients.[10] However, UV light is a very powerful oxidant-promoter which can over-ride antioxidant protection.[11] While antioxidant nutrients are extremely effective in protecting us against more general oxidant exposure, the harsh effects of direct sunlight are best avoided altogether. Chapter 9 goes into detail on how to optimise your antioxidant protection; for more about the sun and skin cancer, see Chapter 14.

SUPER-SENSITIVITIES

Burning and ageing are just two of the negative effects of the sun. UV rays can also cause harm by suppressing the function of the skin's immune cells – the Langerhan cells. In some people, they trigger a reaction which is often mistaken for prickly heat or an allergic reaction to sun cream, called polymorphic light eruption (PLE). Prickly heat is actually a rash which develops when the sweat glands over-react to heat and humidity, as opposed to sunlight.

It is also important to be aware that certain chemicals and medications can increase the skin's sensitivity to ultraviolet light. These include:

- Psoralens, natural plant chemicals found in citrus fruits, parsnips, carrots, celery, buttercups, cow parsley, chrysanthemum and fennel.

- Tretinoin (Retin-A), the drug used in the treatment of acne.

- Antihistamines, some antibiotics (e.g. tetracycline), topical arthritis non-steroidal anti-inflammatory drugs (check with your doctor).

- Some cosmetic ingredients such as musk, bergamot and eosin in lipstick.

- Some chemicals used in toiletries such as hexachloraphene.

In summary, to reduce damage to your skin through exposure to the sun:

- Limit your exposure, especially to strong sun between 10/11am and 3/4pm, and especially if you have fair skin, light-coloured eyes and lots of moles.

- Wear clothing that provides protection – such as a hat and a long-sleeved shirt.

- Use a good sunscreen – at least SPF 7, which contains antioxidants.

- Eat plenty of antioxidant-rich foods (see Chapter 9).

- Take an antioxidant supplement (see Chapter 9).

- Check that any medication you are taking does not increase your sensitivity if you are planning to spend time in the sun.

CHAPTER 5

TEENS AND MENOPAUSE – THE CRITICAL YEARS

Hormones have a considerable effect on our bodies, in particular our skin. So it isn't surprising that when your hormonal patterns are changing your skin is likely to do so as well – most significantly at puberty and again, in women, at the menopause.

PUBERTY

As puberty approaches, the pituitary gland buried deep in the brain produces hormones which trigger the release of other hormones, which, in turn, stimulate the body into developing into an adult. Girls grow breasts and pubic hair and lay down female fat; in boys, the penis grows, pubic hair appears, followed by facial and other hair, muscles develop and the voice deepens.

Girls not only produce more of the so-called female hormones progesterone and oestrogen but also some androgens or male hormones. In boys the emphasis is clearly on the androgens, although they too produce some oestrogen.

Women with high levels of androgens will have more hair growth in areas usually associated with men, while in men this situation often causes male pattern baldness (as opposed to hair falling out for other reasons).

Oestrogens affect your sebaceous glands by making them smaller. They also reduce sebum production and make the sebum less oily. Androgens, on the other hand, increase the size of your sebaceous glands and stimulate the production of more sebum, which is why boys, who produce more androgens (such as testosterone) are more prone to acne (see Chapter 11). Testosterone also has the effect of increasing collagen production, which is why men's skin is tougher than women's. Oestrogen, on the other hand, makes skin softer and smoother.

MENOPAUSE

The effects of the hormonal changes that occur in women between the ages of 45 and 55 are well known, certainly to women who have experienced symptoms of menopause, such as hot flushes, weight gain, insomnia, mood swings and loss of libido. All these are due to the reduced production of oestrogen in the body. More subtle, though, are the changes in the texture of the skin and the way it is supported. As we have seen, the changes in hormones play a significant role in the structure of the skin and the substances it secretes. The key difference between pre- and post-menopausal hormone balance is the decline in oestrogen levels. One of the consequences is that a woman's body is more 'open' to the effects of the androgen hormone testosterone (produced by the adrenal glands). These would previously have been 'masked' or 'opposed' by the presence of oestrogen.

The effects of lowered oestrogen on the skin

- **Oil** The 'unopposed' exposure to testosterone stimulates the secretion of more sebum in the sebaceous glands which makes the skin seem more oily. Acne-like spots and other skin irritations can develop.

- **Hair** Also due to the unopposed testosterone, a woman becomes more prone to developing unwanted hair after the menopause.

- **Thinning** Oestrogen increases the rate at which the cells of the epidermis divide and reproduce. As oestrogen declines, so does the reproduction of new cells.

- **Dryness and loss of suppleness** Oestrogen stimulates the production of certain substances (e.g. hyaluronic acid) which keep the skin hydrated, supple and smooth. As oestrogen levels decline, the skin may therefore become dull-looking.

AVOIDING ENVIRONMENTAL OESTROGENS

In order to counteract the effects of menopausal hormonal changes on the skin on your face and the rest of your body, it is important to reduce your exposure to artificial or 'xeno-oestrogens'. These are oestrogen-like chemicals which are present in the environment. Although this may seem like a good thing when the body's natural production of oestrogen is declining, such substances play havoc with our hormonal balance. They also place a burden on our bodies' inbuilt detoxification systems (see Chapter 8).

Many chemicals have hormone-like properties and have been linked to hormone-disruption – affecting menstrual cycles, fertility, sperm formation, etc. Excessive exposure to harmful chemicals is also linked to degenerative diseases such as cancer.

While it is impossible these days to completely avoid chemicals, or 'anti-nutrients', it is a good idea to minimise the amount that you take in or are exposed to. You can do this by, for example, drinking spring or filtered water, buying organic produce, avoiding household chemicals, not smoking, and not using the Pill or HRT.

NATURE'S HORMONE HELPERS

On the other hand, external oestrogen-like substances from plants – known as phyto-oestrogens – can really help the body at a time of hormonal change. Unlike the potentially harmful oestrogen-like chemicals we are exposed to, those in plants can help to counteract the effects of the body's natural decline in oestrogen. There are plenty of hormone-like substances in natural foods. For instance, soya is a particularly rich source, especially two substances it contains called genistein and diadzein. These are now available as concentrated supplements.

Phyto-oestrogens can also minimise symptoms of the menopause, which could explain why Japanese and other Asian women – whose diet is rich in soya – rarely experience hot flushes or other menopausal symptoms.

Despite some recent negative publicity about soya, there is exceedingly strong evidence of a link between low cancer rates and high isoflavone intake (isoflavones are the active ingredients in soya). One criticism of soya is that it contains substances called phytates, which block the absorption of important minerals such as calcium. But most grains, especially wheat, contain phytates. So we would still say that soya is an ideal part of any diet.

Sources of phyto-oestrogens

- soya.

- alfalfa.

- linseeds.

- beans.

- oats.

- fennel.

- celery.

- parsley.

- red clover tops.

- rhubarb.

- herbs such as agnus castus, black cohosh, dong quai, wild yam.

So, in summary, to minimise your exposure to factors which can interfere with hormone balance:

- Drink spring or filtered water.

- Buy organic produce (as much as you can afford and is available).

- Avoid foods containing chemical additives.

- Reduce your intake of fatty foods.

- Minimise exposure of fatty foods (e.g. nuts and cheese) to plastics (use glass, paper, etc for storage instead of clingfilm and plastic bags).

- Wash all fruit and vegetables.

- Don't buy food that has been exposed to exhaust fumes.
- Reduce exposure to household chemicals.
- Don't smoke.
- Don't exercise near traffic.
- Don't use the Pill or HRT.
- Include sources of phyto-oestrogens in your diet.

CHAPTER 6

NAIL SIGNALS

Many of us spend almost as much time and money on our nails as our skin. Our nails are, in fact, an extension of our skin – composed of hard, closely packed, keratinised cells of the epidermis. They provide important protection for the nerve-rich ends of our fingers. They are also helpful in small but useful ways such as enabling us to scratch or pick up tiny objects. Growth – at a rate of about 1 mm per week – takes place in the nail root, as the skin surrounding the root of the nail develops into nail cells.

Healthy nail beds are pink, due to the rich blood supply underneath. Any changes in colour or structure can give clues to underlying disorders, deficiencies or, more obviously, an accident or external exposure to a harmful substance. The following chart lists the nail problems that can arise and the nutritional deficiencies that often cause them.

Nail signs	Deficiency
Fragile, horizontal and vertical ridges	B vitamins
Spoon-shaped (concave), vertical ridges, brittle	Iron
White spots	Zinc
Fungal infection	'Friendly' bacteria

Nail signs	Deficiency
Splitting	Low hydrochloric acid (stomach acid)
Dry, brittle	Vitamin A, calcium
Dry, curved ends, dark, thin, flat	B12
Horizontal white bands	Protein
Hangnails (split cuticles)	Protein, vitamin C, folic acid
Peeling, cracking, splitting	General nutritional deficiency

In summary, to keep your nails healthy and looking good:

- Follow the Clear Skin diet recommended in Chapter 22, including plenty of fresh fruit and vegetables, and foods rich in sulphur and silicon e.g. fish, broccoli, onions and seaweed.

- Take a good all-round multivitamin and mineral supplement daily.

- Ensure that you have adequate protein intake (e.g. yoghurt, fish, lean meat, eggs, soya, nuts, seeds).

- If you suspect you have digestive problems (see Chapter 7), get a digestion aid supplement that contains enzymes and some hydrochloric acid (stomach acid). This is best done under the guidance of a health practitioner.

- Take a supplement of MSM (a special form of sulphur) which has been shown to improve nail health.

- Treat your nails with care – do not use them to pick or scrape and do not expose them to harsh chemicals (e.g. when washing up, wear gloves).

PART 2

BEAUTY IS MORE THAN SKIN-DEEP

....

CHAPTER 7

DIGESTION – THE KEY TO HEALTH

Your skin is a remarkable barometer of your body's health. As such, it is very much affected by how well you are internally. Most of us look a bit pale after one too many parties – and all sorts of other signs of what is going on inside the body show up in the skin, such as a red face when we are hot and sweaty after strenuous exercise, or a rash in response to something we've eaten.

To keep your skin healthy and to slow down the rate at which it ages, it is essential to look at it not just as an outside casing but as a living, changing organ, every cell of which needs optimum nourishment from both the inside and the outside. In this part of the book we focus on looking after your skin from the inside. As we have already seen, an adequate internal supply of antioxidants is important. So also is a healthy digestive tract and liver.

GUT FEELINGS

Many skin problems are linked to digestion. While an insufficient intake of the right nutrients can affect the health of your skin, so can poor digestion and absorption. Some people eat healthy food but, for one reason or another, don't digest it properly and therefore don't get the nutrients they need.

There's also plenty that can go wrong in the digestive tract which, if laid out flat, would cover a small football field. This surface area is what comes between the 100 tonnes of food we consume in a lifetime and our inner world. Only certain chemicals are allowed through, a selection process which is policed by the immune system.

Prolonged stress shuts down this immune function. It's as if the bouncers go on strike. The bouncers are called IgA (secretory immunoglobulin A); they line the digestive tract and their job is to protect us from undesirable molecules. As our IgA levels fall when we're under stress, we lose this immune response. This is one of the factors that triggers allergies, and it explains why people under chronic stress are more likely to develop food sensitivities.

Too much stress both suppresses the immune system and encourages inflammation, setting the scene for gastrointestinal infections and inflammation elsewhere in the body. Eczema and other skin problems involve inflammation. When we react to stress, the body's attention is diverted towards producing energy for fight or flight, and away from normal tasks like digestion and immunity. That is why it is harder to digest food, and why you are most at risk of getting a cold or flu when you're under stress.

Another reason why these 'uninvited guests' get through into the body is that our inner skin, the wall of the digestive tract, becomes too permeable (a condition known as gastrointestinal permeability or 'leaky gut syndrome'). This can be aggravated by an infection, inflammation, bloating, too much alcohol or the use of antibiotics or non-steroidal anti-inflammatory drugs, e.g. aspirin.

Once too many toxins and large molecules start 'gatecrashing' through the digestive tract, the body has to work overtime to detoxify and deal with them. Before long the

SYSTEM INTOXICATION

- pesticides, herbicides, fertiliser residues on food
- food additives
- alcohol, coffee, tea
- environmental toxins
- water impurities
- food allergies
- medications & recreational drugs
- stress

...lead to...

- poor digestion
- lowered immune response (e.g. infections)
- heightened immune response (e.g. allergies)
- bacterial/fungal overgrowth
- 'leaky gut'
- liver overload
...and much more

...lead to...

- 'irritable bowel syndrome'
- allergies
- skin problems
- fatigue
- mood problems
- joint problems
- hormone imbalance
...and much more

SYSTEM BALANCE

- organic, unprocessed, fresh food
- pure water
- fibre
- vitamins, minerals, essential fats
- good stress management
...plus
- digestive enzymes
- beneficial bacteria

...lead to...

- good digestion
- optimum absorption of nutrients
- efficient liver detoxification
- balanced immunity
- balanced hormones

...lead to...

GREAT HEALTH
- high energy
- clear skin
- balanced moods
- rare illness

Figure 3 – System intoxication vs system balance

body's ability to detoxify all the uninvited guests starts to weaken, resulting in impaired liver function. By this stage even the slightest increase in toxins results in a whole host of symptoms such as fatigue, drowsiness, headaches, body aches and inflammation, as well as poor skin condition. For example, when we exercise, our muscles tend to produce a toxic substance called lactic acid which can make us feel a bit stiff the next day. This is no problem normally, but if a person's detox potential is poor even a brisk walk can trigger symptoms. So too could a slightly larger meal than normal, or certain foods (especially those that are hard to digest).

DIGESTING YOUR FOOD

You are not just what you eat; you are what you can digest and absorb. The large food particles which we eat are broken down into tiny food particles that can enter the body – these small particles are on the guest list, so to speak. Carbohydrates are broken down into simple sugars such as glucose or fructose. Proteins are broken down into amino acids. And fats are broken down into fatty acids and glycerol. Or at least that's what *should* happen.

The digesting is actually done by hydrochloric acid in the stomach and digestive enzymes. Each day your body produces around 10 litres of digestive juices; and if you do not produce enough of these juices you will get indigestion. This can manifest as abdominal discomfort, bloating, excessive flatulence and fatigue. Instead of being energised by a meal, you feel tired. Eating more than your body can digest can also bring on these symptoms.

Bacteria in the balance

Inside your digestive tract are 300 different strains of bacteria, weighing nearly 1.5 kilograms, which are essential for your health and vitality. But if you take a course of antibiotics it more or less wipes them out. Of course, there are harmful bacteria too, which you may have encountered on holiday or from food poisoning. Having the right balance of bacteria is vital to digestive health and overall well-being.

The symptoms of an imbalance are much the same as those for indigestion. You could try taking a digestive enzyme supplement with each main meal. If this doesn't help, you may wish to consider increasing your intake of these beneficial bacteria with a supplement of 'probiotics' (e.g. *Lactobacillus acidophilus* or bifido bacteria). Some supplements contain both digestive enzymes and probiotics. This is especially important if you've been doing anything that is likely to have destroyed them, such as drinking too much alcohol or taking antibiotics. This is the vicious cycle that tends to worsen some skin problems such as acne – taking antibiotics for acne creates an imbalance in the gut which can make the acne worse.

UFOs OF THE INTESTINES

More insidious than bacterial imbalances is UFO infestation. Unidentified faecal organisms (or UFOs) are harmful organisms that can take up residence in the digestive tract, such as bacteria, fungi, protozoa and worms. These parasites are far more common than is generally realised. Symptoms of infection can include:

• Abdominal pain and cramps.

• Fatigue.

• Diarrhoea and constipation.

• Headaches.

• Bloating.

• Food sensitivity.

- Flatulence.

- Weight loss.

- Foul-smelling stools.

- Aches and pains.

- Inflammatory gut problems.

- Fever.

This list is by no means comprehensive but it does illustrate how UFO infestation could underlie many health problems, which can ultimately show up in your skin. If you developed symptoms after being on holiday in a 'high risk' area or perhaps after a course of antibiotics, which wiped out your natural defences against other parasites, then UFO infestation is a possibility. This may seem like a far cry from your skin problem, but if your gut – lined by your 'inner skin' – is not working well for any reason, your external skin may well suffer. A clinical nutritionist can advise you – with the help of a stool test – on the best course of action to take if you suspect that a bug in your intestines may be the root of your health problems.

A particularly insidious and relatively common gut infection is due to an overgrowth of the yeast *Candida albicans*. While it is perfectly normal to have some of this yeast in our digestive tracts, it can proliferate – causing tiredness, bloating and other digestive problems, thrush, premenstrual syndrome, loss of libido and skin problems including athlete's foot, ringworm, acne and psoriasis. A healthcare professional can help you determine whether this may be a problem and give you guidance to eliminate it.

LEAKY GUT SYNDROME

Normally healthy foods can also become toxins to the body if they are not digested or absorbed properly. We are designed to digest our food into simple molecules that can readily pass through the digestive tract and into the bloodstream. However, if a person doesn't digest their food properly, or if the gut wall becomes 'leaky', incompletely digested foods may enter the blood. There they are likely to encounter immune 'scout' cells which treat them as invaders, triggering an allergic reaction.

The ensuing battle results in a complex of chemicals that themselves are toxins and need to be cleaned up to be safe. Instead of promoting your energy and general good health (including clear skin), these foods therefore add to your body's toxic burden. Once this burden becames too great, the body can no longer satisfactorily detoxify itself. This must be a consideration in any skin problem, as many involve inflammation and an over-active immune reaction. Again, this is something a clinical nutritionist can work with you on. Detoxification is discussed more fully in the next chapter.

In summary, to keep your digestive system healthy:

- Avoid alcohol or have it infrequently and in moderation.

- Don't take aspirin or any other non-steroidal anti-inflammatory drugs on a regular basis.

- Cut down your intake of wheat, especially yeasted breads. Switch to oat cakes and wholegrain rye bread instead and rice noodles or buckwheat pasta.

- Eat plenty of fibre-rich foods such as wholegrains, root vegetables, lentils and beans.

- Eat fermented foods such as live yoghurt or take a probiotic supplement.

■ Eat seeds and fish. The essential fats they contain are used structurally in the digestive tract, and act as natural anti-inflammatory agents.

■ If you are suffering from indigestion try taking a digestive enzyme supplement with each main meal.

■ If you are suffering from any digestive discomfort, discuss this with your health practitioner who will be able to help you discover the root cause.

CHAPTER 8

....

DETOX FOR CLEAR SKIN

Eating the right food is one side of the coin and detoxification is the other. Although food is essential and enjoyable, the truth is that almost all food contains toxins as well as nutrients, as do air and water. If you are unable to efficiently detoxify substances from what you eat and your environment, your skin is likely to become congested and unhealthy.

Inside our bodies, substances are chemically broken down, built up and turned from one thing into another. A good 80 per cent of this activity involves detoxifying potentially harmful substances. Much of this detoxifying is done by the liver, which is able to recognise millions of potentially harmful chemicals and transform them into something harmless or prepare them for elimination. It is the chemical brain of the body – recycling, regenerating and detoxifying in order to maintain your health.

These external poisons (or exo-toxins) represent just a small part of what the liver has to deal with; many toxins are made within the body from otherwise harmless molecules. Every thought, every breath and every action can generate toxins. These internally created poisons (or endo-toxins) have to be disarmed in just the same way as exo-toxins. Whether or not a substance is bad for you depends as much on your ability to detoxify it as on its inherent toxic properties. For instance, those with multiple food sensitivities are eating the same food as healthy people – they have just lost their ability to detoxify it.

Instead of thinking of certain substances as 'bad' for you, or provoking a reaction, think of them as exceeding your capacity to detoxify them. It's as if your body's metabolism is a fire. Our metabolic fire – the burning of glucose to form energy – burns slowly and generates plenty of smoke, which the liver has to deal with. It's this 'smoke', rather than the substances themselves, that often causes problems.

TESTING YOUR DETOX POTENTIAL

Skin problems are just one sign of poor detox potential. Others include chronic fatigue, multiple allergies, frequent headaches, sensitivity to chemicals and environmental pollutants, chronic digestive problems, muscle aches, autism, schizophrenia, drug reactions and Gulf War syndrome.

After spending years studying the symptoms associated with impaired detoxification potential, Dr Jeffrey Bland from the Functional Medicine Research Center in Gig Harbor, Washington, USA, developed the Metabolic Screening Questionnaire with common symptoms that indicate a low detox capacity. The following detox capacity questionnaire is based on Bland's research.

Check out your detox capacity

Score 1 point for every symptom you occasionally have, and 2 for those you have frequently.

Head	headaches; faintness; dizziness; insomnia.
Eyes	watery or itchy eyes; swollen, red or sticky eyelids; bags or dark circles; blurred vision.
Ears	itchy ears; ear ache; ear infection; drainage from ear; ringing in ears; hearing loss.

Nose	stuffy nose; sinus problems; hay fever; sneezing attacks; excessive mucus formation.
Mouth	chronic coughing; gagging; frequent need to clear throat; hoarseness; loss of voice; swollen or discoloured tongue, gums or lips; mouth ulcers.
Skin	acne; hives; rashes; dry skin; hair loss; flushing or hot flushes; excessive sweating.
Heart	irregular or skipped heartbeat; rapid or pounding heartbeat; chest pain.
Lungs	chest congestion; asthma; bronchitis; shortness of breath; difficulty in breathing.
Digestion	nausea or vomiting; diarrhoea; constipation; bloated feeling; belching; passing gas; heartburn intestinal/stomach pain.
Joints/muscles	joint/muscle aches or pain; arthritis; stiffness or limitation of movement; feeling of weakness or tiredness.
Weight	binge eating/drinking; craving certain foods; excessive weight; compulsive eating; water retention; underweight.
Energy	fatigue; sluggishness; apathy; lethargy; hyperactivity; restlessness.
Mind	poor memory; confusion; poor comprehension; poor concentration; poor physical coordination; difficulty in making decisions; stuttering or stammering; slurred speech; learning disabilities.
Emotions	mood swings; anxiety; fear; nervousness; anger; irritability; aggressiveness; depression.

If your total score is above 25, you may have a detox problem and you should improve your diet.

If your total score is above 50 your detox potential is under par.

If your total score is above 75 you should seek the help of a medical practitioner.

If you have a significant score it's well worth going one step further and testing your detoxification capacity. Fortunately, modern science has developed non-invasive ways to assess your liver's detoxification potential. The test involves ingesting a measured amount of caffeine, aspirin and paracetamol and then analysing certain chemicals that appear in your urine. How these substances are dealt with, and what they turn into, shows how well each aspect of liver detoxification is working. These comprehensive detoxification tests are available through doctors and clinical nutritionists (see Useful Addresses).

DETOXIFICATION – A TWO-STEP PROCESS

These detoxifying mechanisms, mainly situated in the liver, are a complex set of chemical processes or pathways, that can recycle toxic chemicals and turn them into harmless ones, in a process known as 'biotransformation'. Each pathway consists of a series of enzyme reactions, and each enzyme is dependent on a number of nutrients that, step by step, make our internal world safe to live in.

Detoxification can be split into two stages. The first, known as Phase 1, is akin to getting your rubbish ready for collection. It doesn't actually eliminate anything, just packages it in bin sacks, making it easier to pick up. Fat-soluble toxins, for example, become more soluble. Phase 1 is carried out by a series of enzymes called P-450 enzymes. The more toxins you're exposed to, the faster these enzymes must work to pile up rubbish ready for collection. Often, the substances created by the P-450 enzyme reactions are more toxic than before. For example, many are oxidised, generating harmful oxidants (see Chapter 3).

The function of P-450 enzymes depends on a long list of nutrients, including vitamins B2, B3, B6, B12, folic acid, glutathione, branched chain amino acids (leucine, isoleucine, valine), flavonoids and phospholipids, plus a generous supply of antioxidant nutrients (vitamins A, C and E, etc) to deal with the oxidants.

Often a person who has a high exposure to toxins (perhaps due to diet and lifestyle factors or digestive problems) has a

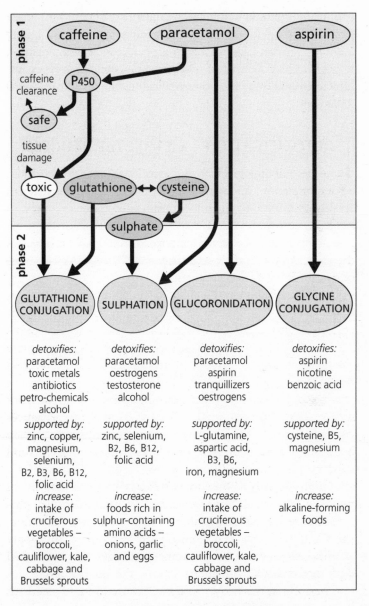

Figure 4 – How the liver detoxifies

revved-up Phase 1, used to working hard and fast to get these toxins ready for collection. Substances that get Phase 1 going include caffeine, alcohol, dioxins, cigarette smoke, exhaust fumes, high-protein diets, organophosphate fertilisers, paint fumes, saturated fat, steroid hormones and charcoal barbecued meat.

The second phase, known as Phase 2, is more about building up than breaking down. According to Dr Sidney Baker, an expert in the chemistry of detoxification, around 80 per cent of all the building that the body does is for the purposes of detoxification. For instance, the end-products of Phase 1 are transformed by 'sticking' things on to them in a process called conjugation. Some toxins have glutathione stuck to them (this is called glutathione conjugation). This is how we detoxify paracetamol (acetaminophen) for example. In cases of overdose, a person is given glutathione to mop up the highly destructive toxins generated by Phase 1 detoxification of this drug.

TOO MANY TOXINS OR NOT ENOUGH NUTRIENTS?

When these biochemical detoxifying mechanisms or pathways don't work properly – either due to overload or a lack of nutrients – the body generates harmful toxins. One example is homocysteine, a toxic by-product of breaking down the amino acid methionine. This can be a result of problems with sulphation (usually a consequence of a lack of vitamin B6), or methylation (which needs folic acid, B6 and other nutrients).

All these detoxifying pathways work together. If one is overloaded, a toxin may be processed by another. But, once the back-up systems are overloaded, the body is unable to clear toxins which can then damage and disrupt just about every system in the body. General poor health, skin problems and a decreased ability to cope with stressors – physical, psychological and chemical – can therefore be a result of an impaired ability to rid the body of harmful toxins, both those taken in from the outside and those generated inside from normal body processes.

In summary, to protect your detoxification capacity:

■ Answer the questionnaire on pages 44–5. If your score is above 30 consider seeing a clinical nutritionist and having a comprehensive detoxification test.

■ Include 'detox-friendly' foods in your diet, for example, green vegetables, onions, garlic, and plenty of other antioxidant-rich foods (see Chapter 9).

■ Eat organic produce.

■ Avoid substances which place a heavier burden on your detoxification capacity, such as alcohol, cigarettes, food additives and non-essential medication.

To find out more read *The Holford 9-Day Liver Detox* by Patrick Holford and Fiona McDonald Joyce (published by Piatkus).

CHAPTER 9

....

SKIN SAVIOURS –
UNDERSTANDING
ANTIOXIDANTS

As we saw in Chapter 3, oxidation is a key factor in the ageing process and general degeneration of skin (as well as the rest of the body), and antioxidants are essential in order to keep this damage in check. Many substances act as antioxidants and the body also has its own elaborate antioxidant defence systems.

In the last decade more and more research has confirmed that many common diseases are associated with a deficiency of antioxidant nutrients and can be eased (or avoided) by taking antioxidant supplements. These include Alzheimer's, cancer, cataracts, cardiovascular disease, diabetes, hypertension, infertility, macular degeneration, measles, mental illness, periodontal disease, respiratory tract infections and rheumatoid arthritis. So, by giving yourself optimum antioxidant protection, you can slow down your visible ageing and also reduce your risk of developing degenerative diseases (which are, in effect, accelerated ageing of a particular part of the body).

ANTIOXIDANTS IN AGEING

Slowing down the ageing process is no longer a mystery. In longevity studies the best results have consistently been achieved by giving animals low-calorie diets, high in anti-oxidant nutrients (in other words exactly what they need and no more). This reduces 'oxidative stress' and ensures maximum antioxidant protection. Animals fed in this way not only live up to 40 per cent longer, but they are also more active. Although long-term human studies have yet to be completed, there is every reason to assume that the same principles apply to us. Already, large-scale surveys show that the risk of disease and premature death is substantially reduced in those with either high blood levels of antioxidants or high dietary intakes of antioxidants. The main players are vitamins A, C and E, plus beta-carotene (the precursor of vitamin A that is found in fruits and vegetables), the minerals zinc and selenium, plus glutathione, lipoic acid and Co-Q10. Their presence in your diet, and their levels in your blood, may prove the best indicator of your power to delay death and prevent disease.

WHAT IS AN ANTIOXIDANT?

Oxygen is the basis of all plant and animal life. It is our most important nutrient, needed by every cell every second of every day. Without it we cannot release the energy in food to drive all our physical processes. There is one problem though – oxygen is chemically reactive and highly dangerous. In normal biochemical reactions oxygen can become unstable and capable of 'oxidising' neighbouring molecules. This can lead to cellular damage which may trigger cancer, inflammation, arterial damage and ageing. So this equivalent of 'nuclear waste' has to be disarmed and neutralised (see Chapter 3).

Oxidation occurs in all combustion processes, including smoking, exhaust fumes, radiation, fried or barbecued food

fried food
burnt/browned food
cigarette smoke
drugs
air pollution
sun light
radiation
toxic industrial chemicals
viruses and bacteria
intense exercise
energy production in our cells
poor liver detoxification

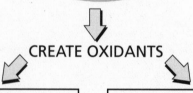

CREATE OXIDANTS

which either
DAMAGE CELLS
which leads to

cancer
heart disease
inflammation
ageing

or are disarmed by
ANTIOXIDANTS

vitamins A, C, E
beta-carotene
bioflavonoids
cysteine
glutathione
co-Q10
lipoic acid
selenium
zinc
copper
B vitamins
countless plant chemicals

Figure 5 – Oxidants and antioxidants

and normal body processes. Chemicals capable of disarming oxidants are called antioxidants. Some are known essential nutrients, like vitamins A and beta-carotene, C and E. Others, though not essential (such as bioflavonoids, anthocyanidins, pycnogenol and many other recently identified protectors found in common foods) are very powerful. Most studies demonstrating the benefits of taking antioxidant supplements, and applying them directly onto the skin, focus on protection from ultraviolet light, but this is only one form of oxidation and the damage limitation goes way beyond that.

We are all constantly exposed to UV radiation (see Chapter 4) and all sorts of other pollutants which age our skin and the rest of our cells. The balance between your intake of antioxidants and your exposure to oxidants determines how quickly your skin and the rest of your body ages. It may also make the difference between life and death. But the good news is that you can tip the balance in your favour by making a few simple changes to your diet and taking antioxidant supplements.

ANTIOXIDANTS WORK IN SYNERGY

None of these nutrients works in isolation in the body, nor are people ever deficient in just one nutrient. It is therefore impossible to underestimate the importance of good all-round optimum nutrition in preventing and reversing the ageing, degeneration and cancer processes.

Vitamin C (which is water-soluble) and vitamin E (which is fat-soluble) are synergistic. Together they can protect the tissues and fluids in the body. What's more, when vitamin E has 'disarmed' an oxidant or carcinogen, the vitamin E can be 'reloaded' by vitamin C, so their combined presence in the diet and the body has a synergistic effect. Research has shown that a combination of vitamin C and E supplements gives people greater resistance to sunburn,[1] while eating antioxidant-rich foods gives us nature's whole spectrum of nutrients, many of which we are not yet aware of.

The same is true of selenium and vitamin E. When these nutrients are provided together, the level of protection they can offer is considerably multiplied. The chart below shows how antioxidants work together to disarm an oxidant. For this reason it is far better to supplement an all-round antioxidant than to just take, for example, vitamin C.

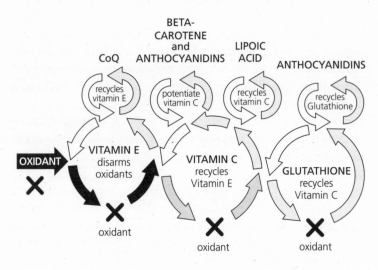

Figure 6 – The synergistic action of antioxidants

VITAMINS A, C AND E

Numerous studies – particularly into UV light – have shown that antioxidant vitamins provide protection from oxidation. Exposure to UV light actually weakens the skin's own antioxidant systems.[2] One study (on mice) showed that the concentration of vitamin C dipped to its lowest 12 hours after being exposed to a single dose of UV light and did not return to its original levels until 72 hours afterwards.[3]

Remember that vitamin C protects the water-soluble parts of cells, while vitamin E is a fat-soluble vitamin. Research showed that vitamin E, when applied to the skin, protected it from the effects of UV light but only when it was applied beforehand or within two minutes, no later.[4] Vitamin A supplementation has been shown to protect the skin from damage caused by UV light.[5] The skin of women taking 30mg of beta-carotene (which the body can convert to vitamin A) did not get as red as those taking a dummy pill, even on parts of the skin covered with sunscreen.[6] In other words, it is crucial to provide your body with the nutrients it needs – both inside and out – in order to prevent oxidative damage in the first place, rather than trying to repair the damage once it has been done.

Beta-carotene is found in red/orange/yellow vegetables and fruits. Vitamin C is also in vegetables and fruits eaten raw, as heat rapidly destroys it. Vitamin E is found in 'seed' foods, including nuts, seeds and their oils, but also vegetables like peas, broad beans, corn and wholegrains – all of which are classified as seed foods. Eating sweet potatoes, carrots, watercress, peas and broccoli frequently is a great way to increase your antioxidant levels, provided, of course, that you don't fry them.

Another great food is watermelon. The flesh is high in beta-carotene and vitamin C. And the seeds are high in vitamin E, and the antioxidant minerals zinc and selenium. You can therefore make a wonderful antioxidant cocktail by blending flesh and seeds into a great-tasting drink.

OTHER ANTIOXIDANT NUTRIENTS

Zinc and selenium

Zinc and selenium are two key antioxidant minerals because they are needed to activate two of the body's main antioxidant enzymes. These are glutathione peroxidase (which is selenium-dependent) and superoxide dismutase (dependent on zinc and, to a lesser extent, copper and manganese). A study done in France showed how zinc and selenium protected DNA (every cell's master blueprint) from oxidative damage from UV light.[7] Seeds and seafood are the best dietary sources of selenium and zinc. Another antioxidant enzyme, catalase, is dependent on iron (although excess iron can also increase oxidation).

Co-Q10

Coenzyme Q10 (or Co-Q10) is not classified as a vitamin because we can actually make it in the body. But Co-Q10 is also a vital antioxidant, helping to protect cells from oxidation and also helping to recycle vitamin E. Co-Q10 works by controlling the flow of oxygen during the cells' production of energy, making the process more efficient. It also prevents damage caused by oxidants formed during the process.

Co-Q is found in all meat and fish (especially sardines), eggs, spinach, broccoli, alfalfa, potato, soya beans and soya oil, wheat (especially wheatgerm), rice bran, buckwheat, millet, and most beans, nuts and seeds.

Glutathione, cysteine and N-acetyl cysteine

The amino acids cysteine and glutathione also act as antioxidants. Cysteine is often supplemented as N-acetyl-cysteine; your body can use cysteine to make glutathione which is the key ingredient in the antioxidant enzyme, glutathione peroxidase, which is itself dependent on selenium. This enzyme helps to detoxify the body, protecting against car exhaust, carcinogens, infections, excessive alcohol and toxic metals. White meat, tuna, lentils, beans, nuts, seeds, onions and garlic are particularly rich in cysteine and glutathione and have been shown to boost the immune system as well as increase antioxidant power.

Anthocyanidins

These are powerful antioxidants from the flavonoid family, found in plants, which account for their different colours. For example, purple, red, orange, yellow and green plants all contain different types of anthocyanidins – so make sure your diet is naturally colourful.

A diet rich in fruits and vegetables can deliver up to a gram of these important nutrients which may be as significant in their health-promoting properties as vitamins and minerals. Anthocyanidins (sometimes called anthocyans) provide dramatic colours in foods such as black grapes, blueberries and cranberries. They are found in fruits, stems, bark, leaves and more specifically in flowers. Grape seeds, bilberries, cranberries and pine bark (pycnogenol) are especially rich sources.

Apart from being important antioxidants, anthocyanidins are also anti-inflammatory which can make them useful in treating or preventing a wide range of inflammatory diseases from asthma to eczema and arthritis. They also help stabilise collagen, our intercellular glue, which protects us against ageing, and keeps our tissue firm, supple and healthy. Remarkably, they provide protection from a wide variety of toxins in both the watery and fatty parts of the body, unlike vitamin C (which protects only the watery parts) and vitamin E (which works only on fat-based compounds).

There are two simple ways to increase your intake of health-promoting anthocyanidins – one is to eat them, the other is to supplement your diet with concentrated extracts. By doing both you will gain the most health benefits. Foods to eat include all sorts of berries, black grapes, citrus fruits, buckwheat and flowers used for herb teas. Drink berry juice and red grape juice (diluted because of its high sugar content) and choose red wine in preference to white.

Lipoic acid

This is a sulphur-containing, vitamin-like substance which has very effective antioxidant properties. It is sometimes known as thioctic acid and plays an important role in the conversion of carbohydrates to energy. As an antioxidant, it is particularly useful because, like anthocyanidins, it is one of the few that is both water- and fat-soluble. This means it can protect a wider range of molecules than, say, just vitamin C or vitamin E. Foods said to be high in lipoic acid are liver and yeast.

ANTIOXIDANT SUPPLEMENTS

Given the unquestionable value of raising your antioxidant status, it is wise to make sure that your daily supplement programme contains significant quantities of them, especially if you are older, live in a polluted city or have any other unavoidable exposure to oxidants.

The easiest way to do this is to take a comprehensive antioxidant supplement, in addition to a good multivitamin and mineral. Most reputable supplement companies (see Useful Addresses) produce formulas containing a combination of the following nutrients – vitamin A, beta-carotene, vitamin E, vitamin C, zinc, selenium, glutathione and cysteine, plus plant-based antioxidants such as anthocyanidins from a source such as bilberry or pycnogenol. The kind of total supplementary intake (which may come in part from a multivitamin and extra vitamin C) to aim for is shown below:

Vitamin A (retinol/beta-carotene)   2500–6600mcg RE (7500–2000iu)

Glutathione (reduced)   25–75mg

Vitamin E   66–660mg (100–1000iu)

Vitamin C   1000–3000mg

Co-Q10   10–50mg

Lipoic acid   10–50mg

Anthocyanidin source   50–250mg

In summary, to increase your antioxidant intake:

■ Include plenty of antioxidant-rich foods in your diet: red/orange/yellow vegetables and fruits such as sweet potatoes, carrots, apricots and watermelon; purple foods such as berries and grapes; green foods such as watercress, kale, alfalfa sprouts and broccoli; 'seed' foods such as peas and wholegrains, fresh nuts, seeds and their oils; onions and garlic.

■ Take a broad-spectrum antioxidant supplement daily.

CHAPTER 10

....

ESSENTIAL SKIN OILS

It may surprise you to hear that fat is good for you. In fact eating the right kind of fat is totally essential for optimal health, as well as good skin tone and avoiding dry skin. Unless you go out of your way to eat the right kind of fat-rich foods, such as seeds, nuts and fish, the chances are that you're not getting enough good fat. Most people in the Western world eat too much saturated fat, and too little of the essential fats, the ones that promote clear, healthy skin.

Saturated and mono-unsaturated fat are not essential nutrients (i.e. you don't need them in your diet), although they can be used by the body to make energy. Polyunsaturated fats or oils, however, *are* essential. Most authorities now agree that, of our total fat intake, no more than one-third should be saturated (hard) fat, and at least one-third should be polyunsaturated oils providing the two essential fats: the linoleic acid family, known as omega 6; and the alpha-linolenic acid family, known as omega 3. (More on these in a minute.) These two essential fat families also need to be in balance, but most people end up with less omega 3 fat in their diets than omega 6.

What's more, these fats very easily become rancid, which is in fact a process of oxidation (as described in Chapter 3). Essential fatty acids (EFAs) react to heat and light – they alter in structure so that they no longer serve any useful purpose in

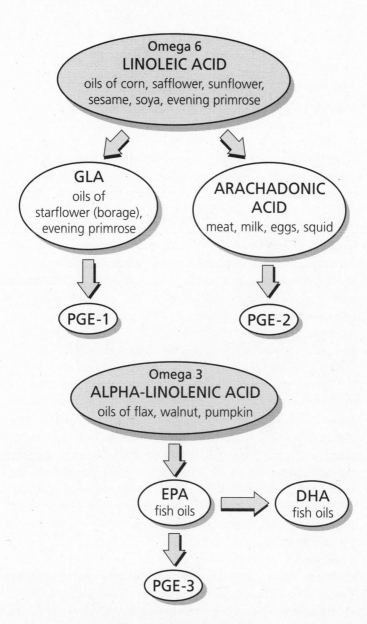

Figure 7 – Essential fatty acids

the body and are called 'trans' fats. In this state they are in fact, quite detrimental to health in that they interfere with the use of EFAs. Many processed foods are deliberately made with such fats precisely because of this alteration in chemical structure which gives them a longer shelf life. So it is important to avoid processed foods which contain trans-fats, as they affect the health of cell membranes, interfere with the liver's detoxification capacity, increase the risk of heart disease, interfere with immunity and many other body processes.

OMEGA 3

The modern diet is likely to be more deficient in omega 3 fats than omega 6 fats simply because the grandmother of the omega 3 family, alpha-linolenic acid, and her metabolically active grandchildren, EPA (eicosapentaenoic acid) and DHA (docosahexaenoic acid), are more unsaturated and more prone to get damaged in cooking and food processing. EPA and DHA can be made into series 3 prostaglandins (PGE-3), which are extremely active hormone-like substances.

We can see this increasing complexity as we move up the food chain. For example, plankton, the staple food of small fish, is rich in alpha-linolenic acid. Carnivorous fish, like mackerel or herring, eat the small fish who have converted some of their alpha-linolenic acid to more complex fats. The carnivorous fish continue the conversion. Seals eat them and have the highest EPA and DHA concentration, then Eskimos eat the seals and benefit from the ready-made meal of EPA and DHA from which they can easily make the series 3 prostaglandins.

These prostaglandins are essential for proper brain function, affecting vision, learning ability, coordination and mood. They also reduce the stickiness of our blood and are used in controlling blood cholesterol and fat levels, improving immune function and metabolism, reducing inflammation and maintaining water balance. Symptoms of deficiency include dry skin, inflammatory health problems, water retention, tingling in the arms or legs, high blood pressure or high triglycerides, infections, poor memory and learning problems, lack of coordination, impaired vision and poor growth in children.

The best food source for omega 3 fats is fish, flax (also known as linseed) and chia seeds. Flax and chia seed oils are less powerful than fish oil (which is rich in EPA and DHA) because they have to be converted into these by the body. Therefore, you need relatively more to achieve the same effect. In practical terms you need a tablespoon of flax or chia oil, which is also available in capsules as a supplement. Supplements usually provide 500 or 1000mg of the oil, with 14g being equivalent to what you would get from a tablespoon of the oil or six tablespoons of flax seeds.

Fish and fish oils provide more powerful sources of the omega 3 fats, EPA and DHA. Eating fish or their oils bypasses the first two conversion stages of alpha-linolenic acid, to provide EPA and DHA. This is why fish-eaters like the Japanese have three times the omega 3 fats in their body fat than the average American. Vegans, who eat more seeds and nuts, have twice as much.

While cod liver oil has the greatest percentage of omega 3 fats, the best fish to eat are more oily fish such as mackerel, herring or salmon. An ideal daily intake of omega 3 fats is about 500–1000mg, or double that if you have an inflammatory health problem, cardiovascular disease or a related mental health problem. This is equivalent to eating 100g of fish three or four times a week. Alternatively, you can take a supplement of fish oils containing EPA and DHA. A good-quality cod liver oil supplement provides 400mg. The most concentrated supplements provide 700mg per capsule. If you had arthritis, for example, you'd need to take three such capsules a day.

Since not all products list their nutrients in the same way the easiest way to measure what you are getting is to look at the label and add up the total amount of EPA plus DHA and compare it to these recommended levels. About half of the omega 3 fats in fish come from EPA and DHA. It is also worth choosing brands and products that are 'PCB-free'. Unfortunately our oceans, and consequently fish, are polluted with these industrial chemicals. Fish oils can be purified to be PCB-free. But not all supplement companies choose such purified oils because it increases the cost. Choose those that do (see Useful Addresses).

OMEGA 6

The grandmother of the omega 6 fat family is linoleic acid. Linoleic acid is converted by the body into gamma-linolenic acid (GLA). GLA then gets converted into DGLA (di-homo gamma linolenic acid) and from there into prostaglandins. The particular kind of prostaglandins made from these omega 6 oils are called series 1 prostaglandins. These keep the blood thin, relax the blood vessels, lower blood pressure, help to maintain water balance in the body, decrease inflammation and pain, improve nerve and immune function, and help insulin to work which is good for blood sugar balance. And this is only the short-list. As each year passes, more and more health-promoting functions are being found. Prostaglandins themselves cannot be supplemented as they are very short-lived. Instead we rely on a good intake of omega 6 fats from which the body can make the prostaglandins we need.

Deficiency signs include high blood pressure, PMS or breast pain, eczema, dry skin, dry eyes, inflammatory health problems such as arthritis, diabetes, multiple sclerosis, mental health problems and excessive thirst.

This family of fats comes exclusively from seeds and their oils. The best seed oils are hemp, pumpkin, sunflower, safflower, sesame, corn, walnut, soybean and wheatgerm oil. About half of the fats in these oils comes from the omega 6 family, mainly as linoleic acid. An optimal intake would be about 1 dessertspoon per day, or 1 tablespoon of ground seeds. Evening primrose oil and borage oil are the richest known sources of GLA. By supplementing these directly you need take in less overall oil to get an optimal intake of omega 6 fats. The ideal intake is probably around 150mg of GLA a day or double this if you have a related health problem. This is equivalent to 1500mg of evening primrose oil, or 750mg of high-potency borage oil (probably about a capsule a day). Most evening primrose oil capsules come in 500mg strengths, giving 50mg of GLA. Therefore you would need to supplement three to six capsules to achieve optimal amounts.

FATS FOR CLEAR SKIN

As you can see, these two types of fats have much to contribute to healthy skin. Each cell membrane – in effect the skin of each cell – is partly composed of essential fats, and your skin is made up of countless such cells. So the fatty acid content of your cell membranes is vital. The fatty acids keep cell membranes smooth and soft and this means that the membranes do a better job of controlling what goes in and out of the cells. When they contain insufficient fat they are not able to retain water, and lose their plumpness.

Many scientists have shown in experiments that if they create EFA deficiencies in animals, the health of their skin deteriorates: they get dehydrated; their skin becomes itchy, dry and inflamed; they are more likely to get skin infections; wounds heal more slowly; the capillaries in the skin become weak and the sebaceous glands become enlarged.[7] As explained above, EFAs also help to reduce inflammation, maintain good blood flow, hormone balance and much more.

In summary, to ensure an adequate intake of essential fats:

- Include plenty of essential fat-rich foods in your diet such as fish, nuts and seeds and their oils. Have seeds in salads or ground up, on cereals, yoghurt or soups.

- Only eat fresh nuts and seeds. Store them and their oils in light- and air-tight containers to prevent rancidity.

- If you have any of the symptoms of an EFA deficiency described above, take an EFA supplement.

PART 3

SKIN SOLUTIONS

CHAPTER 11

ACNE

Spots – every teenager's nightmare and, increasingly, many twenty- or thirty-somethings' hell too. Most of us get the odd spot now and then, but acne can be a long-lasting, painful condition. It can also cause great distress and undermine our self-confidence. Acne is the most common skin complaint. As many as one in two people get it, and of those, a small percentage suffer from serious, ongoing spots which get very infected and leave scars.

Acne affects parts of the skin where there are hair follicles and active sebaceous glands which produce oils or sebum (i.e. mainly on the face, back and chest). It shows up as blackheads, whiteheads and redness due to inflammation. The most common type is *acne vulgaris*, characterised by inflamed, pus-filled spots which open out on to the skin. *Acne conglobata* is more severe – when the infection does not actually break through the skin but stays underneath, forming a painful cyst.

WHAT CAUSES ACNE?

There are various factors which differentiate acne from ordinary spots. The fact that more boys than girls suffer from acne and that people with no male hormones (eunuchs) do not suffer at all gives us some insight into its causes. The amount of the male hormone testosterone in the body increases at puberty (in girls too, although not as much as in boys). This triggers the production of sebum and keratin. Remember that keratin is the main constituent of the epidermis; and an excess of keratin can block pores, as can an excess of sebum. It has now been found that it is not just the increase in testosterone – which happens to all teenagers – but excess conversion to an even more powerful version of the hormone called DHT (dihydrotestosterone) which may bring on acne.[1]

With the increase in keratin, a blockage forms, which in turn creates a build-up of sebum behind it and shows up as a blackhead. As the pore becomes blocked, it provides an ideal breeding ground for the bacteria *Proprionibacterium acnes* which normally lives harmlessly on the surface of our skin. *P. acnes'* ideal party environment is one with no air and plenty of sebum to feed off – so it is easy to see how they have a field day and create an infection in the skin, causing the inflammation and soreness of a spot. If this inflammation gets out of hand, it can spread through to deeper tissues. And, if it does not break through to the surface, it causes a cyst under the skin.

It is also important to note that acne-like spots can be caused by exposure to industrial materials such as mineral oil and coal tar derivatives, sensitivity to certain cosmetics and certain drugs including steroids. So if you are getting spots which seem to be acne, you should first check that they are not being caused by a chemical you are exposed to.

The effect of our hormones on our skin is, obviously, beyond our control. There are, however, other factors over which we can have some influence. The difficulty lies in the fact that there are many factors which must be considered. The link between diet and acne, for example, remains very controversial – some swearing that avoiding chocolate helps, and others finding no relief from giving it up. The best advice is to ensure an all-round healthy diet which includes plenty of fresh vegetables and fruit, wholegrains, some protein (in the form of fish, lean meat, soya products and beans or lentils), and little or no sugary, processed and fatty foods – in fact, the diet described in more detail in Chapter 22. There are a couple of very important things to take into consideration, and one is sugar.

The sugar connection

While many people say that giving up chocolate doesn't cure acne, most of us – not just acne sufferers – find we feel better all round when we give up sugary foods and drinks (see Chapter 22). The connection between sugar and acne is demonstrated by clinical studies which have shown that people who have acne do not process sugar well in their bodies. Insulin is the hormone which helps shift sugar (glucose) out of the bloodstream and into cells where it is used to make energy. People with diabetes either do not produce glucose or do not respond to it, and acne has actually been described by two scientists as skin diabetes.[2] In other words, some people with acne do not transfer sugar into their cells properly.[3]

In order to avoid this, it is important to cut out all sugary foods and drinks, including sweets, chocolate, fizzy drinks, biscuits, cakes, desserts and any added sugar (such as in tea or on cereal). To improve the way the body processes glucose, take 200mcg of the mineral chromium twice daily.

The gut connection

In Chapter 7 we saw how the health of the intestines can have far-reaching effects on the rest of the body. Acne is no exception to this rule, I'm afraid. In fact naturopathic doctors earlier this century considered acne to be a result of a build-up of toxins in the colon. One study showed that half the people with severe acne had higher than normal levels of bowel toxins in their bloodstreams.[4] This usually happens when the bowels are not emptied regularly because of a sluggish digestive system and constipation, which can be caused by a diet low in fibre and fresh foods and high in refined, sugary, fatty foods (e.g. toast with jam for breakfast, a cheese sandwich for lunch, then pizza for supper). Even if a person does not feel constipated, unless they are emptying their bowels properly at least once a day, a build-up of toxic material inside the intestines is likely. We need to get rid of this stuff, otherwise toxins can be reabsorbed back into the body. Think of a sewer system which has nowhere to flow to, with all the build-up and leakage that would ensue.

Another problem for acne sufferers is that they are often prescribed antibiotics to calm their inflamed spots. Although this usually does the trick by reducing the inflammatory effect of the bacteria in the spots, the antibiotics also kill all the important 'friendly bacteria' in the digestive system. This sets the scene for an overgrowth of so-called 'unfriendly bacteria' and other organisms which can release toxins into the body and create all sorts of havoc, including skin problems.

Another factor to consider is sensitivity to dairy products. Cut all milk products out of your diet for at least four weeks and see if that makes any difference.

The Milk and Insulin Connection

Increased sebum production is associated with increased levels of the insulin-like growth hormone (IGF-1). Consumption of dairy products increases IGF-1 levels, as does a high glycaemic load (GL) diet composing of lots of fast-releasing carbohydrates. Eating a low GL diet with no sugar and less carbohydrates and avoiding, or at least minimising, dairy products often makes a big difference.

Stresses and strains

Adult acne, in people who have never suffered from it before, is becoming increasingly common. For many it just appears to come out of the blue, while others get it in their teens and never seem to 'grow out of it'. Nobody knows why so many more people are getting acne later in life but it has been linked to stress. We know that stress interferes with the body's usual hormonal balance. So if you are or have recently been under a lot of pressure, and you are suffering from acne, it is crucial to get the stress sorted out before you can expect to see much improvement. Take gentle exercise such as swimming, walking, yoga or t'ai chi and, if you feel the need, find someone you can talk to about how you are feeling. Another reason why this is so important is that, if you are feeling very self-conscious about the state of your skin, you are likely to get caught in the vicious circle of stress. This will make your skin worse which in turn will make you feel worse and more stressed out.

TREATING ACNE

From the inside

Given that some of the most drastic medical treatments for acne involve powerful forms of vitamin A, it makes sense to include a good dose in your daily supplement programme. Moderation, however, is key, as too much vitamin A (like most substances, even ones that are 'good for you') can be toxic. An ideal level is 25,000iu daily, which you could get from your multivitamin formula. (Women with any chance of getting pregnant should not have more than 5000iu daily.)

Healthy skin also requires a good supply of zinc. It is no coincidence that most acne sufferers are teenagers who are most likely to be deficient, as most of their zinc resources are going into their growth spurts. Zinc is also linked to vitamin A, helping to control inflammation and skin repair. Low zinc levels are associated with increased conversion of testosterone to DHT (see above). An ideal intake is around 45mg a day.

Deficiencies in essential fats (see Chapter 10) have also been linked to acne. These fats are crucial to the health of the skin, its cell membranes, hormonal balance and much more. Taking 1000mg of linseed oil three times a day and/or a source of GLA, such as evening primrose or borage oil, should help. And you should make sure that your diet includes fish and seeds. Vitamin B6 deficiency is particularly associated with acne that is linked to a woman's menstrual cycle. So, in such cases, taking 25mg of B6 three times daily can help.

From the outside

As well as looking after your internal state of health, what you do to the outside of your face matters a great deal too. Because the blocking of pores is a major factor in acne, it is important to keep your face well cleansed and free from clogging oils. Many people make the mistake of over-cleansing their skin, stripping off its natural protective layer of oils. This makes things worse by encouraging the body to produce even more oil and leaving the skin without its natural protection from pollutants and bacteria.

Many 'spot creams' contain benzoyl peroxide – an antiseptic which effectively helps control the growth of bacteria but can also make the skin very dry and sore, so it is important only to use it directly on the spot. 'Less is more' with benzoyl peroxide – just dab a bit on the spot, no more than twice a day, and stop as soon as the spot starts to heal.

Another important factor in the cream – which should contain no more than 5 per cent benzoyl peroxide – is its other base ingredients. Steer clear of substances such as lanolin, D and C dyes (coal tar) or isopropyl myristate, which clog the pores. The prescription cream tretinoin (Retin-A), the acid form of vitamin A, is effective for many people. But it too is pretty harsh as it actually works by peeling away the skin, in effect leaving it about one-third of its usual thickness. As a very last resort, a dermatologist may prescribe isotretinoin (Roaccutane) which, again, can be remarkably effective in calming severe acne, but can also have some serious side-effects such as scaling and thinning of the skin, visual disturbances, nausea, headaches, mood changes, menstrual irregularity and drowsiness.

Tea tree oil – an extract from the Australian plant *Melaleuca alternifolia* – is an effective antibacterial substance and has been shown to be a valid alternative to benzoyl peroxide in treating acne, with fewer of the side-effects such as dryness, scaling and itching.[5] However, very concentrated tea tree oil can itself cause reactions and should not be applied 'neat' to the skin; though it is available in many skin washes and antiseptic creams.

Wash your face with a pH-balanced cleanser, i.e. one that has a similar pH level to the skin (between 4.5 and 5.5). This means avoiding medicated soaps and alcohol toners which make the skin feel very dry, and ultimately stimulate it to produce more oil. Triclosan is a good antibacterial ingredient to look for. It's used in toothpaste, which is where the old wives' tale that toothpaste can help spots may come from.

Whatever you do, don't trick yourself into believing that you do not need a moisturiser – you need a good barrier to keep the skin well hydrated (as opposed to 'oiled') and protected from pollution and the elements. But do make sure it does not contain the clogging substances mentioned above. Some contain 'microsponges' which help absorb excess oil.

Picking or squeezing spots is not a good idea, as this often introduces infection and can leave a scar.

In summary, to avoid or control acne:

- Follow the Clear Skin diet recommended in Chapter 22.

- Eat plenty of fresh, whole foods, including lots of foods that are naturally high in fibre.

- Drink six to eight glasses of spring or filtered water daily.

- Avoid processed, fatty, dairy and sugary foods.

- Try to minimise the amount of stress in your life.

- Make sure you are getting at least 5,000mcg of vitamin A (unless pregnant), 30mg of zinc and 200mcg of chromium daily.

- Use pH-balanced cleansers.

- Use a light moisturiser.

- Use creams containing tea tree oil or benzoyl peroxide very sparingly and only directly on the spots.

CHAPTER 12

....

ACNE ROSACEA

The name *acne rosacea* is rather misleading, in that the condition is not actually related to classic acne, or *acne vulgaris*. Rather, it is a chronic inflammation and swelling of the blood vessels in the skin, which brings on flushing, pimples and sometimes acne-like eruptions on the face.[6] Usually your cheeks and nose are affected but your forehead and chin can be too. Unfortunately, though, it is poorly understood and researchers have been unable to pinpoint its cause.

When it first starts, rosacea usually occurs as intense blushing. If this goes on, the blood capillaries in the skin can break and stay red permanently. In some people, the skin swells and thickens; if this happens around the nose, it may become bulbous in what is known as rhinophyma (as in some people with alcoholism, who often suffer from rosacea). Some sufferers also find that their eyes sting and feel gritty. Rosacea can come up as pustules on the face, which is why it is often confused with acne. It can cause a great deal of discomfort and, because it affects the face, it can also be very distressing and undermine the sufferer's self-confidence.

Rosacea is actually a relatively common skin problem. One in twenty people suffer from it to varying degrees, though many may never realise that they have it. About three times as many women have it as men. It mostly affects people between the ages of 30 and 50 and appears to be more common in fair-skinned people.

NO KNOWN CAUSE

The underlying central cause of acne rosacea is not known, although many factors which seem to bring it on or make it worse are those that encourage the dilation of blood vessels. It has been suggested that a large proportion of people with rosacea produce excessive sebum (the substance which lubricates the skin and keeps it from drying out), although some research suggests otherwise.[7]

Current practice – clinical research to back it up dates back to 1920[8] – has shown that many people with rosacea do not produce enough stomach acid (hydrochloric acid or HCl) and find that their symptoms improve when they take HCl supplements with meals. Indeed, the fact that many sufferer's symptoms get worse when they are stressed bears this out, as stress usually interferes with the production of HCl in the stomach. There is also evidence that people with rosacea do not produce enough of the enzyme which helps digest fats – pancreatic lipase – and that they can reduce their symptoms by supplementing this.[9]

Other research studies have shown that rosacea is also sometimes linked to a deficiency in the B complex vitamins.[10] A small skin mite called *Demodex folliculorum* has been associated with rosacea but most studies have failed to show that it causes the condition or is particularly significant in bringing on the symptoms.[11] One Finnish study did suggest that the mite may be involved in creating the inflammation associated with rosacea.[12] Interestingly, in an old research study from 1940, rats that were deficient in vitamin B2 (riboflavin) were susceptible to infection from *Demodex*, while those with good nutritional status were not.[13]

Factors linked to acne rosacea include:

- consumption of alcohol, hot liquids or spicy foods.

- exposure to sunlight or extreme temperatures.

- skincare products and make-up containing alcohol.

- stress.

- vitamin deficiencies (especially B vitamins).

- low stomach acid.

- low digestive enzymes (lipase).

TREATING ACNE ROSACEA

The usual medical treatment is antibiotics, either taken orally or in the form of topical creams or gels, e.g. tetracycline and metronidazole. This does appear to help control blushing as well as to reduce the inflammation in veins. However, as explained in Chapter 7, antibiotics can provide an immediate solution, but they may have to be used for a prolonged period. This disturbs the beneficial bacteria in the gut and, in any case, does not deal with the underlying situation.

From the inside

Many sufferers of rosacea manage to work out which foods and drinks trigger or worsen their symptoms. The main ones to avoid are: alcohol, coffee, hot drinks, spicy foods and any-thing else which obviously causes the flushing. It is also important to look into gut function – secretion of HCl by the stomach and lipase by the pancreas. Both of these are essential for good digestion. While low HCl is not a direct cause, it is often linked to rosacea.

If you suffer from any of the symptoms shown below, you are likely to be low in HCl and should consider supplementing it. HCl supplements should be taken with main meals. Because of the link between stress and reduced HCl secretion, it is important to relax when you have your meals. And, if necessary, you should take other measures to minimise your stress level such as exercise or relaxation techniques.

Symptoms of insufficient stomach acid include:

- heartburn.

- indigestion.

- feeling of fullness in the stomach.

- feeling hungrier after eating.

- bloating.

- excessive gas.

- bad breath.

Symptoms of low lipase production are similar to those of low HCl but the most obvious way to check for low lipase secretion is how you feel after eating fatty foods. If you have trouble digesting them, then it is possible that you are not producing enough lipase. Again, supplements of lipase, or various digestive enzymes in the same capsule or tablet, can be taken with each meal. It may be necessary to experiment in order to find the best combination of supplements for you.

From the outside

Because of the suspected link with excess grease and the skin mite *Demodex*, it is important to have a good skincare routine which keeps your face clean and protected from sun, wind and cold. Harsh cleansers which contain alcohol, or any which increase the blood flow to the face, are not recommended. Avoiding rapid temperature changes (where possible) also helps reduce the stress on the capillaries of dilating and constricting quickly. Pure aloe vera, which is available in a gel, can ease the burning sensation. And if the redness is more or less permanent, a good make-up base can help camouflage it.

In summary, to avoid or control rosacea:

- Follow the Clear Skin diet recommended in Chapter 22.

- Avoid alcohol, coffee, spicy foods and any others which you know aggravate your condition.

- Take a high-potency B complex supplement, providing at least 100mg of each vitamin.

- Experiment with taking HCl and/or lipase supplements with your meals.

- Keep your skin cleansed and protected.

CHAPTER 13

SKIN HEALING

If your skin is damaged in any way – such as a cut, a graze, a burn, a spot or a surgical scar – a remarkable sequence of events takes place to heal it. A paper cut, for example, is usually gone the next day, while a playground graze heals secretly beneath a scab. Sometimes a cut heals more slowly than at other times, though it's noticeable how quickly most children are left with barely a scar after a nasty graze on the knee. For this regeneration to take place well and quickly, we need a range of nutrients.

HOW DOES A WOUND HEAL?

When the skin has been injured, cells in the epidermis break away from the base, enlarge and move across the opening until it is entirely covered. There appears to be a mechanism which makes them stop moving when they encounter a similar cell, so this migration automatically stops once the surface of the wound is well covered. While this is happening other cells divide and replace those that have migrated across the open space. Then the cells that have formed the new 'skin' themselves multiply to thicken the new surface.

However, if a wound goes deeper into the skin, the process is more complicated. The first step involves inflammation. The purpose of this is to increase the blood supply to the damaged area so that any microbes, or other foreign bodies that may have got into the skin, as well as dead cells, can be taken away. During this stage blood clots are also created around the broken skin to loosely seal the edges. In addition the swelling and inflammation provide a speedier delivery of immune cells which round up any microbes and other cells to help the clotting process. The clot then forms a scab to cover the wound, while the cells beneath can travel across the gap to continue the healing.

In the next stage the cells multiply dramatically so that the damaged blood vessels grow back and collagen fibres form. Once the epidermis underneath the scab is back to its normal thickness, the scab can fall off. A scar may remain where the wound was – if it goes beyond the original skin damage it is what is known as a keloid scar. The difference between normal tissue and scar tissue is that scar tissue is more densely packed with collagen.

WHAT DETERMINES THE PACE OF WOUND HEALING?

The process of healing skin is quite remarkable – all that activity, and sometimes in such a short space of time. Of course, the more extensive or the deeper a wound, the longer it will take to heal but other factors are also important in determining how efficiently our skin cells multiply and mend. As we age, our cell multiplication slows down. But, that aside, nutritional factors play an important role – wound healing is, in effect, growth and repair, processes which require nutrients.

Cell replication and the growth of collagen are essential for damaged skin to repair itself. As in all body processes, a full range of nutrients is needed but the key ones are:

- **Vitamin C** – an antioxidant; also needed for collagen formation.

- **Zinc** – needed for cell replication for healing.

- **Vitamin E** – an antioxidant; helps reduce inflammation and reduce scarring.

- **Vitamin A** – an antioxidant; needed for skin growth and healing.

- **Vitamin B complex, especially B6** – needed for cell replication.

TREATING WOUNDS

It is therefore important to make sure that you are eating a wholesome diet (as described in Chapter 22) in order for rapid healing to take place. You may also want to apply some vitamin E oil or aloe vera gel directly to the skin to speed up the healing process, reduce inflammation and minimise scarring. Vitamin E also helps to reduce inflammation because of its antioxidant properties. Undiluted vitamin E oil is best – if you cannot find it in a bottle or roll-on, break open a capsule, rather than using a vitamin E cream, which will contain other substances.

If there is any sign of infection, diluted tea tree oil in warm water gently poured or wiped over the wound can help fight this. It is obviously important to keep a wound well covered, certainly in its initial stages, to keep out any infection. Any serious burns or cuts, especially those that are slow to heal, should be seen by a doctor.

Many clinical studies have shown that the herb Gotu kola (*Centella aslatica*) helps skin to repair in a variety of situations – from surgical scars to ulcers and external injuries. The active ingredients in Gotu kola are triterpenoid compounds called asiatic acid and asiaticoside. They enhance the basic structures deep in the skin which support collagen, thereby helping the repair of connective tissue and promoting blood flow to the damaged area. Use a source that is standardised to contain 70 per cent triterpenoids and take 30mg of these three times daily.

TREATING BURNS

The healing of a burn is, in effect, similar to that of any other wound and needs the same nutrients and care. The most remarkable healing I have seen in myself was a burn I got on my leg when I had a fall from a motor scooter in Laos. Stopping at the nearest village for a bite to eat, I asked for some ice to soothe the burn. A man disappeared and soon returned offering me some freshly cut aloe vera leaves. I rubbed the oozing gel from a leaf on to my burn, to find great relief. Each day I did the same and, to my great surprise, the wound healed quickly and without any trace at all. I now keep an aloe vera plant and a tube of the gel for any burns, cuts or indeed any skin problems.

Serious burns should, of course, always be treated by a medical professional in the first instance.

In summary, to encourage rapid healing of the skin:

- Follow the Clear Skin diet recommended in Chapter 22.

- Keep any wound or burn clean and well covered to protect it from infection.

- Ensure that you are getting a good supply of nutrients from a wholesome diet and take a multivitamin supplement.

- Apply aloe vera gel and/or vitamin E oil to wounds and burns to accelerate healing and minimise scarring.

- Take 30mg three times daily of standardised extract of Gotu kola.

CHAPTER 14

Skin Cancer

The link between skin cancer incidence and sun exposure is far more tenuous than we have been led to believe. Did you know, for example, that the closer you get to the Equator, the lower is the incidence of cancer? Sunlight, it appears, is both good for you and bad for you. On the one hand, there is evidence that light-skinned people exposed to strong sunlight have more skin cancer. As many as 40,000 Britons get some form of skin cancer annually, although most are non-melanoma (i.e. not fatal). On the other hand, there is some evidence that people deprived of natural sunlight, spending many hours in artificial lighting, may actually have a higher cancer incidence.

THE GOOD NEWS AND THE BAD NEWS

Natural sunlight does generally boost immunity and improve health. (For a fuller discussion of the health effects of light, try reading *Daylight Robbery* by Dr Damien Downing, see Recommended Reading.) One major reason for this could be that exposure to sunlight stimulates vitamin D synthesis in the skin. Although the mechanism by which this may happen is not yet clearly understood, vitamin D has been shown to slow down the proliferation of some cancer cells.[14] This confirms evidence that patients with advanced breast cancer who have high vitamin D levels have a better chance of survival. It may also help to explain why the breast cancer incidence is lower in sunnier parts of the world. Interestingly, natural sunlight actually stimulates cell growth but not during exposure or the first hour thereafter.[15] So we have an hour's grace to mop up oxidants and repair any DNA damage, in readiness for the burst of increased cellular activity following exposure to sunlight.

However, there is a limit to the benefits of sunshine, especially if you are fair-skinned (Chapter 4 looks in more depth at the effects of sun on the skin). People with fair skin (low in melanin), who burn easily and rarely tan when they sunbathe, do have a higher risk of skin cancer when exposed to the high-energy UV radiation of the sun. As research continues, it seems to be becoming more and more evident that it is the combination of a certain skin type with excessive sun exposure that increases the risk of cancer. Other research has, however, shown that genetic factors, such as the number of moles a person has or their natural skin colour, can be more important in determining cancer risk than the amount of time they spend exposed to the sun.

Melanoma risk factors

Most skin cancer, although quite common, is easily treated and rarely fatal. However, about 2 per cent of all skin cancers are of a more insidious nature and are likely to metastasise quickly (i.e. spread to other parts of the body). These are known as melanomas.

If anything, the evidence seems to indicate that inherited characteristics, rather than just sun exposure, may play a greater part in the incidence of melanoma. Some experts also think that just one big, blistery burn as a child can increase risk as an adult, perhaps by damaging the skin's immune cells.

Since 1935 the risk of developing melanoma has increased

twenty-fold. Dr Marianne Berwick, of the Sloan-Kettering Cancer Center in New York, found that those with a large number of moles or with red or blond hair and lighter-coloured eyes or with pale skin had a risk six times higher. However, the rapid increase in incidence does suggest that factors other than genetics are involved. Greater UV exposure (due to changes in holiday habits) and ozone layer depletion are two obvious candidates.

PROTECTING YOURSELF FROM THE SUN

The combination of fair skin, excessive exposure to strong sunlight, and alcohol or smoking is definitely bad news. During strong sunlight exposure there is a high risk of oxidant damage to the skin (that's what burning is). Meanwhile, smoking introduces oxidants into the lungs and bloodstream. Alcohol suppresses the immune system, weakening the body's natural defences. This is also a particularly bad time to be eating a lot of fried or burnt food.

Instead, when you are exposing yourself on some sunny beach, you should use a sunscreen that contains antioxidants. Also, eat plenty of antioxidant-rich foods, such as fresh fruit and vegetables. These high-antioxidant foods are exactly those found in parts of the world where the sun shines long and strong. So nature protects you if you go local. In fact, a report by the World Cancer Research Fund states, 'The chief causes of cancer are tobacco and inappropriate diets.'[16] And it goes on to say, 'Between 30 and 40 per cent of all cancers are preventable by feasible, and appropriate diets and by physical activity and maintenance of appropriate body weight.'

Blocking the rays

External protection is important too. Sunscreens do their job by absorbing UV energy before it gets through to your skin. There are two kinds of UV rays: UVA, an excess of which depresses the immune system and is more associated with age-ing and less with cancer; and UVB, which causes sunburn and damage to skin cells and can initiate cancer. Ideally, you want to limit exposure to both, since UVA can weaken the immune response vital for dealing with damaged cells. (For more on sun cream protection, see Chapter 27.)

The Australian motto is 'slip, slap, slop' – slip on a shirt, slap on a hat, and slop on some sunscreen, especially if you're fair-skinned.

Checking moles

Melanomas start from moles so it's a good idea to check for any changes in moles, especially on the feet, genital folds, breasts, armpits and scalp. Any mole that bleeds, changes its size, shape, colour, texture or sensation should be checked out by a doctor. If malignant melanoma is caught early, there is a 90 per cent chance of recovery. However, if melanomas go undetected for six months this type of cancer is often fatal.

In summary, to guard against skin cancer:

■ Follow the Clear Skin diet recommended in Chapter 22.

■ Minimise the amount of time you spend in strong sun-light, especially if you have fair skin, light-coloured eyes and lots of moles.

■ Use a good sunscreen that contains antioxidants, not lower than SPF 7.

■ Eat plenty of antioxidant-rich foods, especially fruits and vegetables (see Chapter 9).

■ Take a broad-spectrum antioxidant supplement contain-ing vitamins A, C, E, beta-carotene and selenium.

CHAPTER 15

....

PSORIASIS

Psoriasis is one of the most common skin complaints. There are many different types, but it usually appears as clearly defined red patches covered in fine silvery scales. These patches can affect small or large areas of the body, and can be very distressing – not only because they are sore and itchy but also because they can make you feel very self-conscious. Psoriasis is not infectious, and it may be helpful to point this out to anyone who is afraid they might catch it from you. Apart from causing you physical discomfort and loss of self-confidence, psoriasis doesn't actually make you feel unwell.

In the UK, about 2 per cent of the population gets psoriasis – that's more than a million people. It affects women and men equally and it can come on at any age. There appears to be a family link to psoriasis as about one-third of sufferers have relatives with the condition.

WHAT CAUSES PSORIASIS?

Psoriasis is due to a build-up of skin cells that have divided too quickly – in other words, abnormal skin growth. You may remember, from Part 1, that skin develops by means of layers of cells pushing up towards the skin's surface as new ones are made below to replace them. Usually the outer cells are shed so slowly that we barely notice. But in people with psoriasis, new cells are formed about a thousand times more quickly than usual due to a disturbance in the body's cell replication control mechanisms.

Types of psoriasis	Areas it affects	Typical symptoms
Chronic plaque psoriasis (or *psoriasis vulgaris*)	Scalp, knees, elbows or other body crevices	This is the most common type. It causes scaly, red patches which can be very small or cover large areas
Flexural psoriasis	Body crease such as elbows, armpits and under the breasts	Reddening of the skin but no scales
Guttate psoriasis (or teardrop/raindrop psoriasis)	All over the body except for palms and soles	This usually follows about a week after a throat infection. It causes teardrop-shaped scaly patches. It can be completely eradicated if treated early or go on to become chronic plaque psoriasis
Pustular psoriasis	All over the body	Painful pustules which can be accompanied by fever and may come on in response to over use of strong steroids
Erythrodermic psoriasis	All over the body	Very rare. Much of the skin is red, scaly and inflamed, which affects body fluid balance and temperature.

The sufferer's nails are affected by most types of psoriasis. They can become thick, pitted and cracked and may lift from the nail bed.

Some women find that their psoriasis clears up when they are pregnant or reach menopause, so there may be some hormonal link but this is not yet understood. One research study in Denmark found during post mortems that people with psoriasis had overgrown cells which produce the Human Growth Hormone in their pituitary glands.[17] The researchers therefore proposed that psoriasis could be caused by this. In fact, the reason why psoriasis happens at all is not known but there are many ways in which it can be helped.

TREATING PSORIASIS

A key factor in dealing with psoriasis does appear to be managing the way you react to stressful or irritating situations. Indeed, I know of one health practitioner who is reluctant to do any nutritional therapy unless the person with psoriasis is first willing to confront and deal with stress or unresolved emotional issues.

Evaluating stress levels and looking for ways to reduce these or to cope with them better is important in any case, but particularly in a chronic condition such as psoriasis. This may take the form of dealing with an issue directly, talking to a therapist, doing a personal development or stress management course, or taking up t'ai chi or yoga (see Useful Addresses) – whichever course of action feels most appropriate for you. Other therapies such as reflexology or aromatherapy, when carried out by a qualified practitioner, can also be very relaxing (see Useful Addresses).

From the outside

Traditional medical treatment usually involves using emollients to moisturise the skin, or coal tar preparations which are messy and smelly. Harsher chemicals such as dithranol are relatively effective. But they are also messy, can stain the skin and harm normal skin, and are too strong to be used on the face, groin or armpits. Other treatments include salicylic acid, retinoids, steroids and vitamin D. While these can all be very helpful, they are not without side-effects, such as severe skin irritation; and ultimately, they do not get to the cause of the problem. More radical treatments, using powerful drugs such as methotrexate, help stop cell growth, but these are quite toxic and affect all cells in the body.

Ultraviolet light therapy is a very useful treatment for people with psoriasis (although in a very few cases it can make it worse). Substances such as psoralens, which increase the skin's sensitivity to light, are often used in conjunction with light therapy. Because of the risk of skin cancer with ultraviolet exposure, this only tends to be used as a last resort and has to be carefully monitored.

Natural sunlight and bathing in the sea can be very helpful. Indeed, visiting the sunny shores and waters of the Dead Sea is a popular therapy for people with psoriasis, if rather expensive. A cheaper alternative is to put a kilogram of Epsom salts and 500 g of salt in a warm bath, or even one of the Dead Sea products which are available in healthfood shops. You may also want to look in your local healthfood shop for alternatives to cortisone creams such as glycyrrhetinic acid (made from licorice) which can be just as effective, or camomile or cayenne pepper extract (capsaicin).

From the inside

As with many skin problems, there seems to be a significant link between gut health and psoriasis. External treatments will never cure the condition until the internal cause is dealt with. Balancing the mechanisms which control skin cell division appears to be vital, and these mechanisms can only function properly when the digestive tract is working well. If the lining of the intestines is not healthy – due to constipation, poor digestion, food allergies or whatever – toxins can get into the body and affect the skin.

Enzymes

One of the main gut problems in people with psoriasis appears to be faulty digestion of protein; this, in turn, creates excessive toxicity in the bowel, which weakens the gut lining and allows substances to intoxicate the rest of the body. This can lead to skin problems including psoriasis and other forms of inflammation.

Taking a herbal mixture called Swedish bitters can stimulate the digestion, and a digestive enzyme supplement taken with each main meal should also help. The body naturally produces proteolytic enzymes (which digest protein) but may not be producing enough, so taking a source of these may help. Look out for a formula containing protease – the broad name for enzymes which digest protein. Bromelain is an extract from pineapple, available in supplement form, which does this.

Herbs

Toxins produced in the body by undesirable bacteria or yeasts such as *Candida albicans* (see Chapter 7) in the intestines can affect the compounds which control cell division. However, the herb sarsparilla can bind to toxins and clinical studies have shown it to help people with psoriasis.

Other herbs which can help cleanse the digestive tract are oregon grape, which was traditionally used in chronic skin conditions such as psoriasis (or goldenseal which has some similar properties), and oregano, which is also a powerful detoxifier. You may, with the help of a herbal practitioner, want to follow a bowel-cleansing programme of specific herbs and fibres such as pectin or psyllium.

Any build-up of toxins also has the knock-on effect of burdening the liver, the body's main detoxification organ. The liver usually filters out toxins from the gut before they get out around the body, but if it is overloaded it becomes less efficient at this. The herb milk thistle (*Silybum marianum*) helps support the liver, as does the mineral sulphur. This can be increased in the diet by eating more eggs, onions and garlic and can be taken in the form of MSM supplements – 1000mg, three times a day.

Diet and supplements

It is therefore important to have a diet which supports good digestive and liver health – high in whole foods that are naturally high in fibre such as wholegrains, root vegetables, lentils, fresh fruit, fresh vegetables (especially green ones) and beans. You should also avoid foods that have a negative effect on the gut and liver, such as fats, alcohol and sugars in particular, as well as any foods that may be acting as irritants (most commonly wheat and dairy products). Eliminating these two food groups from your diet should only be done with the guidance of an experienced health practitioner.

In addition to eating a healthy diet and checking for food sensitivities, people with psoriasis can benefit from supplementing particular nutrients to promote the health of the skin and calm inflammation. Vitamin A (up to 5,000mcg daily) and the mineral zinc (up to 30mg daily) are essential for good skin health. Quercetin is a plant bioflavonoid which has powerful antioxidant properties and can help soothe inflammation – take 400mg three times a day. Large doses of vitamin C (i.e. more than 500mg a day) should be avoided. There are many essential nutrient supplements that may be beneficial, but taking those above and a multivitamin is a good way to start, in addition to some essential fats.

It's important to limit animal fats from meat and dairy

products because they can promote inflammation, as can commercially processed foods (e.g. margarine or foods containing hydrogenated fats) and fried fats which also interfere with the way the body processes essential fats. Conversely, fish oils and other essential fats can help control inflammation. Eat fish such as salmon, mackerel or herring at least three times a week; and have fresh pumpkin and other seeds daily. If you can get hemp seeds or linseeds, grind them in a coffee grinder and sprinkle them on cereals, soups or salads; use cold-pressed pumpkin, safflower, sunflower and other oils on salads or on food after it has been cooked (heating these oils damages them). Also, each day take either a dessertspoon of flax seed oil, or a fish oil supplement which provides at least 1000mg of EPA. Sprinkling lecithin granules on food can also be beneficial, as it helps with the body's use of fats.

Interestingly, one clinical study found that psoriasis patients tended to be deficient in protein and folic acid due to the extremely rapid growth of their skin cells, which created extra demand for these nutrients.[18] While it is not necessarily recommended that people with psoriasis dramatically increase either of these nutrients, this does underline the need for a good diet.

Unfortunately, finding out what best keeps your psoriasis at bay is often a question of trial and error. Go for those methods which do not involve large financial outlay first, as what works for some may be of little use to others.

In summary, to avoid or control psoriasis:

■ Follow the Clear Skin diet recommended in Chapter 22.

■ Eat plenty of fibre-rich foods.

■ Take supplements which promote detoxification of the bowel and liver.

- Eat foods rich in essential fatty acids, and supplement fish oil or flax seed oil.

- Promote good protein digestion with the use of Swedish bitters, and digestive enzymes at mealtimes.

- Avoid or limit your intake of animal fats from meat and dairy produce.

- Avoid or limit your intake of alcohol and sugary foods and drinks.

- Detect and eliminate any foods which may be irritating your gut.

- Take measures to reduce and manage stress and unresolved issues in your life.

CHAPTER 16

....

ECZEMA AND DERMATITIS

The name eczema is derived from a Greek word meaning 'to boil'. As such, it describes an inflamed, red rash which is usually intensely itchy. In more severe cases, the skin is broken and becomes weepy and scabbed. Even in people who have managed to control their eczema the tell-tale signs – of toughened, red skin with exaggerated furrows around the eyes and neck – speak of a condition that may now be under control or 'outgrown' but once caused severe discomfort.

Also known as dermatitis, eczema comes in several forms – atopic, seborrhoeic, contact and others. Dermatitis usually refers to a skin condition brought on by a reaction to something outside the body. So, contact dermatitis, as its name suggests, is triggered by exposure to particular substances such as detergents or certain metals. Seborrhoeic dermatitis tends to affect oily areas of the body such as the scalp and face and is not normally so itchy. The word eczema is usually used for conditions which are not caused by external irritants. The National Eczema Society estimates that one in ten people has eczema at some time in their lives.

Atopic eczema is usually regarded as a hereditary condition, often associated with asthma, hay fever or urticaria (hives, see Chapter 18) in the same person or his/her family. It is said to affect up to 3 per cent of the population.

Like many skin problems, conventional treatment for eczema involves the use of creams applied locally. In other words it tends to deal with the symptoms from the outside. Emollients are used to keep the skin soft and lubricated; and corticosteroid creams can be very effective at relieving inflammation and itching in the short term. However, their long-term use is questionable, not only because many users become insensitive to their effects, and therefore need stronger formulas in higher doses, but also because of the side-effects that come with long-term use. Corticosteroids can stunt growth, weaken bones, suppress the adrenal glands and cause many other problems. Ultraviolet light treatment can also relieve the symptoms of eczema, although, again, the dangers that come with it (i.e. the risk of skin cancer) make it a questionable practice.

PHYSIOLOGICAL DIFFERENCES

Several physiological 'weaknesses' have been found in people with atopic eczema. Not only do they generally have more allergies, and a tendency to get hay fever and/or asthma, but they also tend to have some sort of disordered fat metabolism which makes their skin dryer and less able to hold moisture. There is also an increased likelihood of an abnormally high amount of the bacteria *Staphylococcus aureus* in their skin.

In addition, people with eczema have been shown to have abnormalities in their immune system, causing certain cells to release higher amounts of histamine and other allergic compounds, which in turn cause inflammation and itching. Studies have also shown another immune system abnormality which results in an inability to kill bacteria effectively. All of these factors put together – resulting in itching, scratching, broken dry skin and susceptibility to infection – give us a clearer understanding of how eczema symptoms, and the accompanying severe discomfort, arise. They also give a clearer indication of how they can be alleviated.

Food allergies

Unfortunately, many eczema sufferers only turn to nutritional therapy once emollients and steroid creams have become ineffectual in alleviating their condition. Yet there is increasing evidence that even atopic eczema may be triggered or at least exacerbated by food-related reactions. Despite the apparently genetic nature of atopic eczema, many people with eczema find considerable relief when they follow a diet that avoids some common food allergens and many practitioners see the identification and elimination of these as a primary treatment strategy. Indeed, Dr Stephen Davies writes, 'Any child with eczema should be considered to be intolerant of cows' milk and eggs until proven otherwise.'[19]

As with many food allergies, the best treatment is breast-feeding in infancy and prevention by avoidance. If a baby does get eczema while he/she is still being breast-fed, it is often because of an allergic reaction to foods in the mother's diet. One study showed that avoidance of common allergens, such as milk, eggs and peanuts, as well as fish, citrus, wheat, chocolate and soy by the mother helped.[20] If a baby develops eczema at around the same time as they are weaned from breast milk, cows' milk or other recently introduced foods must be suspected. (For more on allergic reactions, see Chapter 18.)

The best way of diagnosing a food allergy is to avoid common allergens such as milk/dairy produce, gluten, eggs, fish, food additives and peanuts for at least ten days. These foods should then be reintroduced, one at a time, at five-day intervals to check for any reaction. Unfortunately, the main milk alternative, soya, can also be highly allergenic. One investigation identified milk, eggs and peanuts as the cause of 81 per cent of childhood eczema.[21] Research done in Glasgow showed a significant improvement in the amount and severity of eczema after only four weeks in children who avoided eggs compared to those who did not.[22]

Any food must, however, be considered, and any found to bring on a reaction should be avoided for at least a year. Strict avoidance diets should be followed with particular care in children, to prevent any nutrient deficiencies; although, with guidance from a nutritionist, this should not be difficult. Rice, millet, fruit, vegetables and meat can be eaten instead of the allergens and, with some imagination, can make up a tasty, healthy diet. (For more on allergies, see Chapters 18 and 25.)

It is extremely important to identify and eliminate any allergies as these can cause 'leaky gut',[23] in which the gut becomes more permeable to inappropriate food molecules which place yet more strain on an already struggling immune system. This usually leads to further allergies – a vicious cycle of events that can make a sufferer's life quite miserable and also makes it difficult to follow effective elimination diets. Another condition of the gut which has been linked to eczema and other allergic conditions is an overgrowth of the yeast *Candida albicans*. High levels of antibodies to candida have been found in people with eczema; the higher the levels of antibodies, the more severe the eczema patches.[24]

TREATING ECZEMA

As with many health problems, it is important to maintain good gut health in controlling eczema (see Chapter 7). Not only does this minimise the effects of any food sensitivities, but it also reduces the potential burden on the immune system from any poorly digested food or ingested toxins. It is therefore essential to avoid sugar and refined, processed or fried foods. During initial treatment it may be helpful to take a bowel-cleansing formula which supports the liver and pro-biotic supplements (e.g. acidophilus) to ensure a healthy gut environment.

Essential fats

A key factor in controlling eczema is maintaining good mois-ture in the skin. For this, it is essential to have adequate amounts of essential fats in your cell membranes. Many skin diseases are related to faulty metabolism of essential fatty acids (EFAs), although there is some controversy about exactly which fats are involved. Nevertheless the general consensus is that people with atopic eczema have poor function of the delta-6-desaturase enzyme. This leads to a build-up of linoleic acid (an omega 6 fat), as it does not convert efficiently to GLA (gammalinolenic acid). In such a case, supplementing evening primrose, borage or starflower oils (at least 250mg of GLA daily) may be helpful. With children, rubbing the oil from a 500mg capsule directly onto the skin three times daily can provide some relief. One reason why babies sometimes develop eczema when they are weaned is that they are usually switched to a diet much lower in EFAs than their mother's milk, so adding an EFA blend to their food may alleviate this.

Some studies have shown, however, that omega 3 fats are just as effective in controlling eczema, if not more so. One study demonstrated that the ratio of omega 3 fats to omega 6 was lower than normal in people with eczema.[25] In fact most modern diets are much higher in omega 6 fats than omega 3; and the fats are often modified commercially to the extent that they provide little nutritional value and even interfere with proper fat metabolism.

Supplementing EPA and DHA fish oils or even eating 'oily' fish, such as salmon, sardines, tuna and mackerel, regu-larly are efficient ways of incorporating omega 3 fats into your cell membranes, making the skin retain more moisture.

Supplementing linseed oil, also an omega 3 fat, is a cheaper, but less efficient way of doing this, as it must first be converted to EPA/DHA in a metabolic process which depends on a good supply of vitamins and minerals.

In any case, it is always important to include sources of essential fats in your daily diet, largely in the form of oily fish and seeds (pumpkin, sunflower, sesame, hemp and linseed). The first three of these can be eaten as snacks, while the others need to be ground. A mixture may be kept in a glass jar in the fridge and ground daily for use on cereal, salads or soups. Essential oil blends (see Useful Addresses for suppliers) can be used in salad dressings or on food (after it has been cooked).

Supplements

Several nutrients are required for the conversion of omega 3 and 6 fats to their more active forms. These include vitamins B3, B6, C, biotin, zinc and magnesium. A deficiency in any of these will impair conversion and may result in increased inflammation. Zinc is also needed for several components of the immune system, which is likely to be stressed by any food allergies and any infections in the eczema lesions. Indeed, in a 1990 study, children with atopic eczema were found to have low serum zinc levels.[26]

The B vitamins are needed for energy production, which is essential for all good health including healing. Vitamin A is helpful in preventing skin dryness and can be taken orally or used as a skin emulsion. Another fat-soluble vitamin, E, can also relieve dry skin; fat-soluble vitamins help maintain the integrity of the fat-soluble part of cell membranes, thus safeguarding their ability to maintain moisture. You need to ensure an adequate supply of all vitamins and minerals if you have eczema, as any deficiency is likely to manifest itself in the skin before any other organ. (The body cleverly prioritises the organs which are essential for life when it hands out what is available; needless to say, the skin is not high on the list.)

Supplements of flavonoids (plant compounds with powerful antioxidant properties), especially quercetin, have been found to be very helpful in controlling eczema through their ability to inhibit histamine release and their antioxidant activity.[27] Foods rich in flavonoids are citrus fruit, berries, onions, legumes and green tea; while other compounds that contain significant amounts include grape seed extract, bilberry and Ginkgo biloba. These and quercetin are all available in supplement form, either alone or as part of a formula.

Licorice is another herb which has been shown to have significant anti-allergy and anti-inflammatory properties; indeed, it is usually included in Chinese herbal preparations which have become increasingly popular in the treatment of eczema. Creams containing glycyrrhetinic acid from licorice or camomile can be helpful in alleviating the severe itching that plagues eczema sufferers. It is important to do this, not only for reasons of comfort but also because scratching can break the skin which increases the chances of infection by bacteria and ultimate hardening of the skin.

External factors

Many people with eczema soon discover which products aggravate their condition such as certain soaps or creams, detergents, or types of wool. With these, it is mainly a case of detecting which are the worst offenders and avoiding them. Some people simply have contact dermatitis (i.e. the condition only arises in a reaction to allergens such as metals or creams). However, a recent study involving children in Nottinghamshire, published in the *Lancet* in 1998, found that there was also a link between the incidence of eczema and the hardness of water where the children lived.[28]

Many people with eczema also find it helpful to be aware of substances and materials that their skin comes into contact with, such as cosmetics, fabrics, household cleaning products and detergents. Pure cotton clothing is usually less irritating than synthetic fibres or even wool. It is also important to avoid contact with cleaning products – use rubber gloves and products which do not contain harsh chemicals. Many people have found great relief from using a product called eco-balls (see Useful Addresses for suppliers). These are placed inside the washing machine instead of detergent and leave no residue in clothes. Using a mattress cover to minimise contact with dust mites is also helpful for some sensitive people. And for those whose eczema gets worse when they are under stress, it is important to do something to relieve this such as regular exercise or yoga.

So, while eczema is a frustrating, severely uncomfortable condition that affects children and adults alike, there are clearly many ways of dealing with its root causes, without having to resort to medication that merely alleviates the symptoms. Although detecting and eliminating allergens and building the appropriate nutritional status to deal with eczema may take a little time, it can ultimately provide significant, longer-lasting relief.

In summary, to avoid or control eczema:

- Follow the Clear Skin diet recommended in Chapter 22.

- Detect and eliminate any food allergens – most common are milk, eggs and peanuts.

- Have at least three servings of fish a week and take an omega 3 oil supplement (fish or linseed) daily.

- Limit your intake of meat and dairy products.

- Take a flavonoid supplement such as quercetin (300mg before meals) or grape seed extract (50mg with meals).

CHAPTER 17

CELLULITE

'Orange peel' skin causes a great deal of angst for many women. Cellulite, as the 'orange peel' look is more properly known, affects as many as 90 per cent of women, yet it is still regarded with horror, and some people spend a great deal of money trying to get rid of it. Remember the day when newspapers showed close-up, encircled parts of Princess Diana's legs, 'exposing' the fact that she had the dreaded cellulite, and – surprise, surprise – was not the flawless woman many had portrayed her as.

Yes, the rich and famous *do* have cellulite, but it is still something most of us would go to great lengths to smooth out – even though some doctors say it is simply the perfectly normal storage of fat. Unfortunately, there is no magic answer to this problem, and it is not entirely clear why and how it forms in the first place. What we do know, however, is that it is not just found in overweight women and that it hardly affects men. Cellulite is most commonly found in the thighs and buttocks, but can appear on the upper arms, the back of the neck and the abdomen. If it is extensive, it can actually make the affected areas feel heavy and tight. It must not be confused with cellulitis, which is an inflammation of the connective tissue of the skin.

WHAT IS CELLULITE?

Scientists have examined cellulite tissue in great detail to understand what it is and attempt to work out how to get rid of it. The cells involved are in the subcutaneous tissue, the layer just under the surface of the skin, where there are fat cells. In women this layer of fat chambers is deeper, and the connective tissue is thinner than in men. Having said that, these differences apply to the whole body – not just the areas in women most likely to be affected by cellulite.

As women age, the layer of elastic connective tissue in the dermis and the layers between the fat chambers get even thinner and less flexible. When this happens, the fat chambers are not so well supported and can easily become enlarged and misshapen. The actual dimpling of the skin comes about because of the distortion of the fat cells in the subcutaneous layer and the weakening of the connective tissue (which is normally more elastic) between each one (see Figure 8). Examining cellulite areas of skin under a microscope, scientists found that the fat cells protruded up into the dermis in affected areas, but not in normal areas.[29] They also found that the connective tissue was not as smooth and regular in cellulite. The lymphatic system, which permeates all parts of our bodies, also becomes weaker and less efficient as women age. Men don't suffer from cellulite in the same way because they have a thinner layer of fat chambers and stronger connective tissue.

The lymphatic system is an extensive network of vessels which run between all our cells and act as a waste dump – fluids pass into the lymph vessels and are filtered at various points called lymph nodes (the 'glands' in your armpits, groin, neck, etc). The fluids can only enter the lymph and move along its vessels because of the movement of the body (the lymph system is not powered by a pump in the same way as the blood system). The cells of the lymph vessels are attached

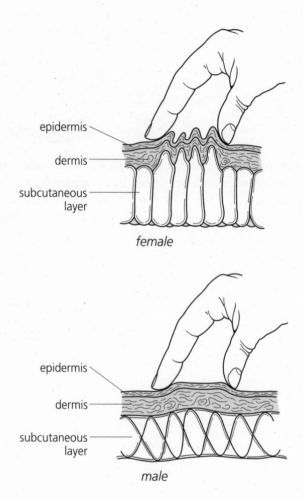

epidermis

dermis

subcutaneous
layer

female

epidermis

dermis

subcutaneous
layer

male

Figure 8 – Skin differences between women and men

to the surrounding cells by collagen and elastin fibres, so physical movement opens up the gaps to allow fluid in and move it along. Saggy collagen and elastin therefore contribute to a sluggish lymph system, which is, in turn, associated with the development of cellulite.

WHAT CAUSES CELLULITE?

Cellulite is actually more of a cosmetic issue than a health condition, although its presence usually indicates some sort of congestion in the body. Simply rubbing on creams or lotions will not make much difference at all – cellulite needs to be seen from the perspective of the whole body, i.e. from the inside.

The exchange of nutrients, waste products and other substances between cells depends on how efficiently the cell membranes select what goes through them, as well as on the efficiency of the blood flow and lymph circulation. When the body is sluggish or overloaded – through poor diet or lack of exercise – none of these processes works well. The result is a build-up of toxins between the cells.

The healthier your body is, the better it is at clearing toxins and burning up fat. The fluid between your cells drains into the lymphatic system, which filters it at the lymph nodes. The lymph may become overburdened with the toxins and this is a significant contributor to the development of cellulite. Women who have persistent cellulite usually have a tendency to be constipated too – another sign of congestion and poor clearance of waste products from the body. Following a really toxin-free diet intermittently (like the one suggested in Chapter 8) significantly reduces the load on your body and allows it to carry out its internal cleansing routine more efficiently.

It's not just fat

Cellulite is not a build-up of fat. Even thin people can have it. The link between fat and cellulite is mainly that enlarged fat cells do put pressure on the connective tissue between the fat chambers, which affects the smoothness and tautness of the skin. Also, if a person is overweight, with large fat deposits, their metabolism will probably be sluggish (not to mention the other health risks of being overweight such as diabetes and heart disease). Keeping the connective tissue strong helps reduce cellulite, so that it is able to keep its shape, even if any build-up of fat does take place.

So, although cellulite isn't the same as fat, exercising and minimising fat build-up do come into any anti–cellulite programme. Exercise is also important because muscle movement stimulates lymph flow as well as blood circulation. Good blood flow will enhance the delivery of oxygen and nutrients to your cells, thereby optimising the way they work and the way they get rid of waste products. Any attempt to lose fat, however, must be done gradually, as rapid weight loss will leave skin saggy, especially in older women whose connective tissue is already thinning due to hormonal changes.

HOW TO BEAT CELLULITE

Ideally, you should avoid getting too much cellulite in the first place. That said, let's get real! If, like many people, you already have some cellulite you need to follow an all-round programme to reduce it: minimising toxin build-up, improving circulation, maintaining an ideal weight and amount of fat, and strengthening your connective tissue. As far as weight loss goes, eating a healthy diet and correcting any other body imbalances you may have with the help of a health practitioner can get you a long way towards helping your body reach its ideal weight. You could also read *The 30-Day Fatburner Diet* which gives detailed guidance on effective, healthy weight loss (see Recommended Reading).

From the outside

Stimulating your, lymph flow is essential, in order to keep what is, in effect, your body's 'waste disposal system' running smoothly. Exercise helps, as does skin brushing, and lymphatic drainage massage (which must be carried out by a trained professional – see Useful Addresses).

To skin brush, get a natural bristle brush, ideally with a long handle, from your local health shop or chemist. Brush your entire body when it is dry, using a dry brush. Go more gently where the skin is more delicate such as on the chest, neck and belly. Start with your feet and work your way up your legs, then brush up your arms towards your chest and across your back. Do this before your morning shower.

Turning the shower to cold at the end, if you can face it, is another way of stimulating circulation. And if you have access to a sauna, a few short bouts (5–10 minutes), with a cold shower in between, is very stimulating and invigorating.

From the inside

The obvious way to avoid a build-up of toxins is to reduce the amount you are exposed to. Diet-wise, this means eating fresh, unprocessed foods, and organic as much as possible. For people who can digest them, raw vegetables are very rejuvenating and cleansing. Avoid all refined, commercially processed foods which are generally low in nutrients and high in additives and fats. Most of us know which foods are 'clogging' – heavy, rich, fatty, stodgy foods should be off the menu. The Clear Skin diet in Chapter 22 gives you some guidelines to follow.

Eating foods rich in nutrients which support the connective tissue can be helpful. For instance, peppers, kiwi fruits, broccoli, citrus fruits, tomatoes, blackcurrants, strawberries and peas are all rich in vitamin C; while cherries, blueberries, blackberries, red grapes and buckwheat are full of bioflavonoids. Certain herbs have also been found to be effective in helping reduce cellulite, probably because they have properties which strengthen connective tissue. For example, several research studies have shown that taking Gotu kola (*Centella asiatica*) orally significantly improves cellulite.[30] It apparently helps to stimulate the basic structures deep in the skin which support collagen, thereby strengthening the connective tissue. The active ingredients in Gotu kola are asiatic acid and asiaticoside. For best results use a source that is standardised so that 70 per cent consists of these acids; take 30mg three times daily.

There is no easy answer to cellulite once it has developed. But exercising regularly to keep fit and boost your circulation, minimising your exposure to toxins, maintaining your ideal body weight, daily skin brushing and eating vitality-laden foods should stop it getting worse, and may, with persistence, even help to reduce it.

In summary, to avoid or control cellulite:

- Follow the Clear Skin diet recommended in Chapter 22.

- Eat plenty of fresh, colourful vegetables and fruits.

- Avoid foods containing additives and chemicals.

- Avoid foods containing sugar and animal fats.

- Exercise at least three times a week.

- Skin-brush daily.

- Take a supplement of Gotu kola – 30mg three times daily.

CHAPTER 18

....

RASHES AND HIVES

If you come up in a rash or hives, the first thing you need to check is whether you are suffering an allergic reaction to something you have eaten or been exposed to. Hives – also known as urticaria – are raised, white welts on the skin, surrounded by redness. The swelling and redness are caused by the release of one of the body's allergy chemicals, histamine. There are many factors which can trigger such a reaction – from a scratch, heat or cold to a number of foods and additives. So the first step towards controlling it is detecting and eliminating the trigger.

WHAT ARE ALLERGIES?

Allergies occur when the body alters its normal immune response in some way, due to the presence of an allergen. Allergens are substances which bring about this immune response in a particular individual.

In sensitive people, the immune cells over-react to these substances. When the offending allergen combines with specific immune cells called antibodies, other cells release granules containing histamine and other chemicals that cause the classic symptoms of allergy – such as skin rashes, hayfever, rhinitis, sinusitis, asthma and eczema. Severe food allergies too, for example, shellfish or peanuts, may result in immediate gastrointestinal upsets or swelling in the face or throat. Such allergies can cause severe, life-threatening reactions.

WHO SUFFERS FROM ALLERGIES?

Cases of allergies are rapidly increasing and are now thought to affect as many as one in three people. But it's not known whether this is due to an overall decline in the competence of our immune systems, an increased burden on them, or perhaps a bit of both. Allergies can sometimes run in families. However, they may not take the same form down the generations. Allergic symptoms can also change with age. A baby with eczema may grow out of it, only to become an adult who suffers from hayfever. (For more on allergic reactions in the skin, see Chapter 16, on eczema.) If you do come up in a rash, it is also necessary to rule out specific disorders such as chickenpox, shingles, rosacea or herpes, which may initially look like a rather nondescript rash.

WHAT CAUSES HIVES?

Physical factors

One of the most common causes of hives is pressure on the skin – often from fabric or jewellery or even another person. Within minutes, sensitive people can come up in welts. Another common cause is heat – which triggers a rash more commonly known as 'prickly heat' and forms as a result of an over-reaction in the sweat glands. It is not only heat from the sun but also from exercising, a hot bath, eating spicy food or even a stressful life event which can trigger this type of rash. In other people, urticaria is brought on by the cold, whether it be cold air, cold water or a cold object.

Reactions to chemicals

The most common cause of urticaria is, however, a reaction to medication – particularly antibiotics (including penicillin) and aspirin. Indeed, some people have very severe reactions to penicillin. Unfortunately, penicillin is sometimes present in foods and drinks such as milk[31] without us knowing.

People with chronic (long-term) urticaria are often sensitive to aspirin. It is possible that, in addition to triggering a direct reaction, the aspirin creates a vicious circle, whereby the gut becomes more permeable or 'leaky' (see Chapter 7). This in turn makes the immune system more sensitive. If you do come up in a rash or hives when you are on medication, contact your doctor to check whether this may be the cause. If it is, you will both have to decide whether the need for the drugs outweighs the discomfort of the urticaria.

Drugs and other substances which can cause an outbreak of hives

- aspirin
- allopurinol
- antimony
- barbiturates
- bismuth
- chloral hydrate
- chlorpromazine
- corticotrophin
- essential oils
- fluorides
- food colourings
- meprobamate
- mercury
- morphine
- penicillin
- phenobarbitone
- pilocarpine
- polio vaccine
- preservatives
- procaine
- promethazine
- quinine

- gold
- griseofulvin
- insulin
- iodine
- menthol
- reserpine
- saccharin
- salicylates
- sulphites

Reactions to foods

The most common cause of hives in children is a reaction to foods or food additives. The foods which are most likely to bring on urticaria in sensitive children are: milk, fish, meat, eggs, beans or nuts,[32] although any food can do so. Others to consider are chocolate, cured meats, chicken, citrus fruits and shellfish.

However, avoiding suspect foods is only part of the solution. It's also very important to make sure that the digestive tract is working well – that all the right digestive juices are being released, that the gut wall is strong and healthy, and that elimination is taking place regularly. If these processes are not working well, the lining of the gut does not perform its filtering role properly; and the gut's own immune system does not perform its guard duties properly.

Reactions to additives

Our food is increasingly contaminated with chemicals used to colour, flavour, sweeten, stabilise and preserve it. While many of these substances do not produce any visible, negative reactions in most people, they are clearly not a natural part of the human diet, and they place an added burden on our detoxification systems. For some sensitive people, such chemicals are just too much for their immune systems and they come up in an allergic reaction in the form of hives. If a child has any sort of unexplained rash, food additives, as well as certain foods, should be suspected.

Another way in which allergies can show up in the skin is with oedema, or water retention. If you have puffiness or bags under your eyes (or water retention elsewhere) you may be sensitive to a food you are eating such as wheat or dairy products.

One of the most common food additives which causes reactions (including hyperactivity and asthma) is tartrazine, also known as E102, which is used as a dye to colour foods orange and yellow. Interestingly, both tartrazine and aspirin block a reaction in the body which subsequently triggers the production of the body's natural allergic chemicals called leukotrienes. These are even more powerful than histamine. Numerous scientific studies have shown that additive-free diets are very helpful to people with hives.[33]

Eating fresh food, as close to its natural form as possible, is the main way of avoiding the potential hazards of commercially prepared foods. The Clear Skin diet (see Chapter 22) focuses on natural, tasty foods. Having organic food is another way of avoiding added chemicals in both animal and vegetable produce.

An experienced health practitioner will be able to help you identify where the problem lies and tests are available to determine any insufficiencies in the digestive process. You should also seek the guidance of a nutritionist or other professional when following any elimination diet, especially in children, as it is important to have a full range of essential nutrients. (For more on food allergies and the way they trigger reactions, see Chapters 7 and 16.)

TESTING FOR ALLERGIES

Testing for allergies is notoriously difficult. There are numerous allergy tests available, each claiming to be accurate. But trials have shown that such tests can produce widely varying results. Some are, however, reasonably accurate, especially in detecting particular types of allergies.

Skin prick test

In this test a drop of allergen is put on the skin, which is scratched to allow the allergen to enter the body. Inflammation indicates a positive response. This is good for direct skin-related allergies but not so accurate for inhalant or food allergies.

RAST

For the RAST (radioallergosorbent test) serum is separated from a blood sample and then placed on samples of allergens. If the serum contains antibodies to that allergen, a complex is formed. The level of sensitivity can also be measured. This is the most accurate test for immediate allergic reactions, rather than slower reactions; and it is more likely to pick up food allergies than skin tests.

ELISA test

The ELISA (enzyme linked immuno sorbent assay) test also uses blood serum to test reactions to various allergens, and can test for more subtle, slower reactions and levels of sensitivity.

Avoidance testing

Perhaps one of the most accurate ways of discovering allergens is for the sufferer to avoid suspect foods for a time and then watch for any reaction when they are reintroduced into the diet. It is important to do this with the guidance of an experienced practitioner, as suitable alternatives (which provide a full range of nutrients) must be eaten.

Foods that provoke an immediate response usually have to be avoided for life. Others that produce a more delayed reaction may be reduced or avoided for some time. It is generally best to avoid suspect foods for at least a month, then test. After long-term avoidance (up to six months) it is unlikely that any 'memory' of a reaction to that food will remain.

Another option, after a strict, one-month avoidance, is to 'rotate' foods so that each food is only eaten every four days to reduce the build-up of allergen-antibody complexes. (For more on avoidance testing see Chapter 25.)

TREATING ALLERGIES

Anti-allergy nutrients

Vitamin C is a natural anti-histamine which can often alleviate symptoms of an allergic reaction such as hives. Not only does it help reduce the release of histamine, but it also helps the body break it down more quickly. Take 1–3g during the course of a day.

In nature, vitamin C is usually found alongside substances called bioflavonoids – one of these, quercetin, has been shown to also help reduce the inflammatory reaction. Take 200mg three times a day.

Foods which contain vitamin C include peppers, peas, kiwi fruits, broccoli, citrus fruits, tomatoes, blackcurrants and strawberries. Some companies make special blends of anti-allergy nutrients (see Useful Addresses for suppliers).

Coping with stress

Many people find that they react to stressful events with a skin rash or hives. For instance, I knew a woman who always wore a neck scarf when she had to deliver a public speech because her neck came up in scarlet bumps when she was nervous. Stress triggers all sorts of changes within our bodies, including a reduction in our immunity, which may well be behind this reaction. In such cases, dealing with stress by means of relaxation or resolving a stressful situation is important, especially if the hives become chronic. Yoga, meditation, relaxation tapes (see Useful Addresses) or, for a more long-term problem, perhaps counselling could be helpful.

In summary, to avoid or control rashes or hives:

- Follow the Clear Skin diet recommended in Chapter 22.

- Detect and eliminate the cause of the rashes or hives – avoid suspect external factors, foods and all food additives.

- Boost the body's own natural anti-inflammatory processes with vitamin C (2g daily) and a bioflavonoid such as quercetin (200mg three times daily).

- If stress triggers the hives, try to do some sort of daily relaxation.

CHAPTER 19

....

COLD SORES

Cold sores actually have very little to do with a cold or even the cold weather. They are recurrent clusters of small blisters which form a red, weepy patch usually around the mouth or lips which usually turns into a scab. The patches are very contagious so hands must be washed after contact with the blisters and contact with others should be avoided. You should also be careful about sharing cutlery, towels, lip balm, or indeed anything that may have touched the sore.

WHAT CAUSES COLD SORES?

These sores are caused by the Herpes simplex I virus. The cold sore is likely to develop around a week after you have been exposed to the virus, although some people seem to be immune, even when they do come into contact with it. The first sign of developing a cold sore is a tingly, sore feeling with a small bump which then turns into a blister. The lymph nodes or 'glands' in the area may become sore and swollen too.

Once a person has had a cold sore, the virus remains dormant in the body and usually resurfaces at times of stress, which lower resistance. The stress may be due to emotional upheaval, lack of sleep, poor diet, overindulgence in alcohol, an infection elsewhere or exposure to the sun. Some women find that outbreaks are linked to their menstrual cycle. So once the virus is in your body, keeping your immune system strong is vital in order to avoid an outbreak or at least minimise your risk of one.

The same virus and a similar one called Herpes simplex II can cause genital herpes. The symptoms are similar, but in the genital region, and you may feel unwell or a little feverish. The same 'no contact' advice applies and, of course, includes having safe sex.

TREATING COLD SORES

It is possible to reduce outbreaks of cold sores by eating a diet high in the amino acid (protein constituent) lysine and low in arginine. Doing this on an ongoing basis can help reduce the likelihood of an outbreak. And you should certainly follow this diet as soon as you feel a cold sore developing. Research

Foods high in arginine	Foods high in lysine
Avoid or minimise:	*Increase*:
• Peanuts	• Fish and shellfish
• Other nuts	• Turkey and chicken
• Chocolate	• Vegetables and fruit
• Seeds	• Beans (not soya)
• Cereals and grains (e.g. oats, rye, corn)	• Beansprouts
• Gelatine	
• Soya	

has shown that the Herpes virus needs arginine to reproduce itself, while lysine blocks the replication. During an outbreak, it's a good idea to take L-lysine supplements, although it should not be taken continuously for long periods of time (i.e. more than three months).

Over-the-counter cold sore remedies containing aciclovir (e.g. Zovirax) do the trick of drying out the cold sore effectively. This is perfectly OK once you've got a cold sore, but prevention is better than cure.

Supporting your immune system

The two most important nutrients for boosting your body's resistance are vitamin C and the mineral zinc. You should make sure your usual supplement programme includes at least 1000mg of vitamin C daily and 15mg of zinc. When you get a cold sore, however, increase this to at least 2000mg of C and 45mg of zinc, spread throughout the day, and add 1000mg of bioflavonoids. Research has shown that doing this can shorten the duration of the outbreak.

A cream containing concentrated extract of the herb lemon balm (or *Melissa officinalis*) has been shown to prevent the recurrence of cold sores when it was used during the initial infection.

In summary, to avoid or control cold sores:

- Follow the Clear Skin diet given in Chapter 22.

- Avoid foods rich in arginine and boost your intake of foods containing lysine.

- Eat plenty of garlic, a powerful immune booster.

- Take L-lysine 1000mg three times daily.

- Take vitamin C 1000mg twice daily.

- Take bioflavonoids 1000mg daily.

- Take zinc 15mg three times daily.

- Apply vitamin C and zinc cream or L-lysine cream (see Suppliers, under Useful Addresses) – as directed.

- Use concentrated lemon balm (*Melissa officinalis*) cream as directed, at the first sign of infection.

- Apply ice at the first sign of tingling for 10 minutes at least three times a day.

CHAPTER 20

....

FUNGAL INFECTIONS

Athlete's foot and ringworm are two of the most common infections caused by fungi, although many different types can affect the mouth, the fingernails, the genitals, around the anus, in fact almost anywhere on the body. They are infectious and are mostly found in warm, damp areas such as between the toes (athlete's foot), the groin ('jock itch'), the vagina (thrush), the mouth (also thrush) and can even be the cause of nappy rash in babies. Most fungal infections are very itchy.

Athlete's foot (properly known as *tinea pedis*) thrives particularly between the toes, feeding off the dead skin cells. The symptoms are sore cracks, inflammation and peeling skin. It is highly contagious, particularly in warm, damp places such as changing rooms at gyms and swimming pools. If bacteria get into the cracks, they can become infected and even more painful.

Ringworm is a fungal infection of the scalp or other skin. It takes the form of small red spots that grow to about 1 centimetre across and has nothing to do with worms at all. The middle of the spots starts to heal, leaving rings of red, scaly borders.

Sometimes a breast-feeding mother and her young baby can continually re-infect each other from a nipple infection and oral thrush.

Fungal infection under the nails (*paronychia*) may make the nails discoloured and they can come away from the nail bed.

TREATING FUNGAL INFECTIONS

The most common underlying cause of any fungal infection is lowered resistance, coupled with the destruction of the beneficial bacteria that usually live in our bodies. These bacteria are easily killed by antibiotics and other drugs, not only those we take in directly but also those in our food supply.

So, if you are susceptible to any sort of fungal infection, you should increase your intake of beneficial bacteria by eating live, natural yoghurt and perhaps taking a probiotic supplement such as *Lactobacillus acidophilus* or bifido bacteria, especially if you have to take a course of antibiotics. *Bifidobacterium infantis* are an ideal strain of bacteria for young children. Choose a brand that contains 'billions' of viable organisms per gram (not millions). It will be one that needs to be refrigerated, and don't cut costs because – as with most things – it is likely to be a false economy.

You also need to eat a diet of fresh, unrefined foods and avoid sugar – on which fungi thrive – in order to support your immune system and reduce the risk of the fungus proliferating. Garlic is a strong anti-fungal and immune-boosting agent, so include plenty of that in your diet too.

From the outside

Tea tree oil is a powerful antifungal which can be used externally on infections. Dilute a few drops in warm water and bathe the affected area with clean cotton wool (for ringworm), or soak the area (for athlete's foot or infected fingernails) or gargle in the case of oral thrush – three times a day.

Tea tree oil is widely available from healthfood shops and chemists. A very small number of people are sensitive to it, so try it on an uninfected patch of skin first (diluted). Lavender oil is a suitable alternative. For athlete's foot, vinegar – neat or diluted – makes an effective foot wash.

It is important to create conditions in which the fungus is less likely to take hold e.g. drying carefully between your toes and using unscented talcum powder or Mycota powder to prevent dampness. If, however, you have recurring infections, you should see a health practitioner who will be able to help you detect and rectify any underlying cause, such as low immunity.

Keep affected areas as dry as possible and try not to let them come into contact with healthy skin; wear clean, cotton clothing and underwear and wash towels after each use.

If you are breast-feeding and your baby develops oral thrush or you have pains or discharge from your breasts, contact your doctor or nurse immediately.

In summary, to avoid or control fungal infections:

- Follow the Clear Skin diet given in Chapter 22.

- Avoid sugar in all forms – added to drinks, on cereal, in sweets, chocolates, biscuits, desserts, sugary drinks.

- Eat live, natural yoghurt daily.

- Eat garlic daily.

- Take a probiotic supplement – as directed.

- Bathe the affected area in diluted tea tree oil or another effective antifungal agent.

CHAPTER 21

OTHER SKIN CONDITIONS

FACIAL PUFFINESS

Puffiness, which is usually most noticeable around the eyes, can be due to all sorts of reasons, not least a late night. The puffiness is generally caused by water retention, even if you do not have swelling elsewhere, and this in itself can be brought on by a number of factors. If you find that you have puffy eyes regularly, no matter how well you sleep, it may be worth checking with your doctor that you don't have any underlying problems with your kidneys, bladder or heart, or an underactive thyroid.

Other possible causes of water retention, in the face or otherwise, are:

- **Food allergy/sensitivity**

- **Premenstrual syndrome**

- **Excessive salt intake** – avoid adding salt or eating packaged foods which usually contain it

- **Inadequate water intake** – contrary to what may seem logical, drinking lots of water does not actually increase water retention – it's the body's poor management of water balance that does this

- **Low potassium** – increase your intake of fresh fruit and vegetables and wholegrains

- **Other nutritional deficiencies** such as essential fatty acids (EFAs) or vitamin B6.

If you are prescribed diuretics (which help reduce the water level in the body), it is important to supplement magnesium (400mg daily) because diuretics can cause this important mineral to be lost in the urine. Magnesium and potassium are essential for proper water balance in cells. EFA deficiencies (see Chapter 10) can mean that the skin does not have its ideal 'water-proofing' from the inside, so excess water is lost through the skin.

Natural, diuretic herbs can be helpful – but in the long term it is always best to tackle the root of the problem. In the meantime, make enquiries at your healthfood store. Many companies make blends of herbs aimed at balancing water in the body. These usually contain dandelion, uva ursi, celery seed or solidago (golden rod).

Working out whether or not you are sensitive to any foods is best done with the support of a nutritionist, but you can do a simple (free!) test yourself. The most common sensitivities are to wheat and dairy products, so you could cut each of these out of your diet (one group at a time) for at least three weeks and see if you notice any difference.

For wheat, avoid: bread, pasta, pizza, anything made with pastry, biscuits, cakes, muffins, crumpets – anything containing flour. For dairy, avoid: milk, cheese, yoghurt, ice cream, fromage frais and anything made with milk (e.g. chocolate, creamy sauces, lasagne, Yorkshire pudding). Wheat and dairy products are 'hidden' in many foods. You will soon notice if avoiding (or eating) these foods makes a difference. For more on avoidance testing see Chapter 25.

In summary, to avoid or control facial puffiness:

- Follow the Clear Skin diet given in Chapter 22.

- Rule out any underlying illness with your doctor.

- Eat plenty of fresh fruit and vegetables.

- Do not add salt to your food and avoid packaged foods.

- Drink at least 2 litres of water daily

- Increase your intake of EFAs – have at least three servings of fish a week and take an omega 3 oil supplement (fish or linseed) daily.

- Identify and avoid any foods you are sensitive to.

IMPETIGO

This is a highly contagious skin infection, usually caused by the staphyloccocus (staph) bacteria, or sometimes strepto-coccus. It mostly affects children. The symptoms consist of red lumps anywhere on the body, particularly the face and hands, which become filled with pus and erupt into yellow scabs. Staph bacteria are actually all over the place, including on the skin of most healthy people, so impetigo is only likely to develop if a person's immune system is below par. If this is the case, the bacteria can take hold, causing the infection, so it's clearly vital to eat a diet that supports your immune system.

Good general hygiene and thorough care of any breaks in the skin are both important to prevent infection. Because impetigo is so contagious, it is essential to avoid touching the pustules, to avoid contact with others, and to change your clothes, bed linen and towels daily. Antibiotics may be needed to eradicate the infection, especially if it spreads into the body.

In addition to following a generally health-promoting diet (see Chapter 22), it is essential to cut out sugar intake from any source, be it cane sugar, honey or fruit. (Many bacteria, including staph, feast on sugar and reproduce prolifically.) Important nutrients during such an infection are vitamins A and C and zinc. Garlic is also a powerful natural antibiotic and can be taken in supplement form as well as in food.

Tea tree oil (diluted or in an ointment), applied to the pustules directly, is strongly antibacterial.

In summary, to avoid or control impetigo:

■ Follow the Clear Skin Diet given in Chapter 22.

■ Avoid sugar in all forms – added to drinks, on cereal, in sweets, chocolates, biscuits, desserts, sugary drinks, and also in fruit, fruit juices and honey.

■ Take a garlic supplement and eat garlic daily.

■ Take vitamin A – 25000iu for adults, 10000 iu for children.

■ Take vitamin C – 3000mg for adults, 1000mg for children.

■ Take zinc – 45mg for adults, 15mg for children.

All nutrients are for short-term use only – no longer than two weeks.

LIP PROBLEMS

Sore lips and cracks at the corners of the mouth are usually a sign of a deficiency in B vitamins, or vitamin C. They may also be caused by a deficiency in essential fatty acids (see Chapter 10).

Rather than simply turning to supplements to deal with lip problems, look at your diet. Make sure you are getting a good range of nutritious foods and not taking in too many antinutrients such as alcohol, sugary or refined foods, and foods with added chemicals. Smoking is also a big no-no.

In summary, to avoid or control sore lips:

- Follow the Clear Skin diet given in Chapter 22.

- Take a B complex supplement or make sure your multivitamin contains at least 50mg of each of the B vitamins.

- Take at least 1000mg of vitamin C daily.

- Have at least three servings of fish a week and take an omega 3 oil supplement (fish or linseed) daily.

VITILIGO

Vitiligo is a pigment disorder in which the colouring of the skin is disturbed – the melanocytes (cells which give skin its colour) are no longer able to make melanin. This creates patches of whitish skin – either a couple of small ones or covering large parts of the body – which are extremely prone to sunburn. The hair on the affected area is usually white too. The actual cause is not known, although it sometimes happens after a physical trauma or alongside another disease such as diabetes or thyroid problems.

Vitiligo has been linked to a deficiency in stomach acid (HCl) production, so supplementing this with each meal may help. Some people find that taking B complex vitamins (plus extra B5 and PABA), vitamin C and zinc help improve the condition.

WARTS

These skin growths are caused by one of a number of human papilloma viruses. With the exception of genital warts, they are not generally very contagious between people although they can spread from one part of the body to another. They can occur anywhere on the body but the most widespread are common warts (usually on hands and knees), plantar warts (on the soles, often referred to as verrucae) and genital warts (which can spread to the anal area).

Common warts don't usually hurt but verrucae can make walking painful; genital warts can be very uncomfortable and obviously affect normal sexual activity, not just because of the discomfort but also because they are highly contagious. Although most warts are completely harmless, some that affect the cervix have been linked to an increased risk of cancer. So if you suspect you have genital warts you should see your doctor.

As with any other infection, warts take hold due to lowered resistance, so it's advisable to eat a good diet (see Chapter 22) and avoid foods which deplete your body of nutrients. Deficiencies in vitamins A, C and zinc can also reduce your immune system's strength.

Medical treatment of warts depends on their location. Common warts are usually removed by burning, freezing and other methods, but they often return. A huge range of topical applications have been suggested to get rid of warts, though they are not always successful. Common ones to use, on the affected skin only, are: a thin slice of garlic; Thuja oil or tincture, aloe vera gel, clove oil, vitamin C cream or pure paste of vitamin C powder.

In summary, to avoid or control warts:

- Follow the Clear Skin diet given in Chapter 22.

- Avoid sugar in all forms – added to drinks, on cereal, sweets, chocolates, biscuits, desserts, sugary drinks; also fruit, fruit juices and honey.

- Avoid alcohol, coffee and smoking.

- Take a multinutrient which contains vitamin A and zinc.

- Take vitamin C – 1000mg for adults, 200mg for children.

PART 4

ACTIVE SKIN REJUVENATION

CHAPTER 22

EAT YOURSELF BEAUTIFUL

As we have seen, eating plenty of fresh, untreated foods is essential for the health of your entire body, not just your skin. A good intake of antioxidants is particularly vital (see Chapters 3 and 9), as it reduces the speed at which your body ages and degenerates.

Other dietary factors have been covered in previous chapters, such as keeping your digestive tract and liver in good working order (see Chapters 7 and 8) and the importance of essential fats (see Chapter 10). This chapter outlines some general dietary guidelines and reminds you of the dangers of sugar in your diet.

THE CLEAR SKIN DIET

Having read the information in this book, you may have realised that your digestion is not what it could be, and that this is having a knock-on effect on your skin. In this case, you may want to seek the advice of a qualified nutritionist to take you through a full nutritional programme or any changes you wish to make (see Useful Addresses).

Because of the diverse nature of skin disorders and all the different underlying causes it is impossible to give blanket dietary guidelines which apply to everyone. So below are broad guidelines for an optimum diet, which should be followed in addition to the particular suggestions given in other chapters. Buy organic produce as much as possible.

Dos	Treat with care	Don'ts
Water: Have six glasses each day.	**Alcohol:** Avoid completely or limit your alcohol intake.	**Sugar:** Don't add sugar to drinks and cereals, and avoid sugary foods such as soft drinks, sweets, jams, many cereals, biscuits, cakes and desserts.
Colourful fruit and vegetables: Have five daily servings, including red/orange/yellow vegetables and fruits, purple foods, green foods, onions and garlic, and 'seed' foods such as peas.	**Tea and coffee:** Have no more than two cups a day.	**Refined carbohydrates:** Don't have foods containing white flour, such as bread, biscuits, cakes, pastries and pasta.
Fresh seeds: Each day have one tablespoon of mixed fresh seeds, e.g. pumpkin, sunflower, sesame or ground hemp/linseed.	**Vegetable oils:** Limit vegetable oils to a little olive oil and/or cold-pressed sunflower or other oils.	**Chemicals:** Don't have foods containing chemical additives. This includes most canned, preserved or processed foods.
Essential fats: Have a tablespoon of cold-pressed seed oils daily and oily fish three times a week.	**Red meat:** Limit red meat to no more than three times a week. Have fish, organic chicken or game instead.	**Fried foods:** Don't have fried foods. Boil, steam, bake or lightly grill them instead.
Fibre-rich foods: Eat plenty of wholegrains, root vegetables, lentils and and beans.	**Grain foods:** Limit foods made from wheat, oats, rye, etc. to one or two portions each day.	**Fatty foods:** Don't have foods like butter, cream and ice cream.
Organic foods: Eat organic as far as possible.		**Processed fats:** Don't have processed foods as most of them contain trans-fats.
Alternatives to dairy products: Try sometimes using alternatives to milk and cheese such as soya milk and tofu.		**Smoking:** Don't smoke at all.
Vegetable sources of protein: Include some soya, beans, lentils and sprouted seeds.		
Yoghurt: Have low-fat, live, organic yoghurt.		

Following these guidelines, a day's meals might look like this:

- **Breakfast:** Natural, live yoghurt with chopped fresh fruits and a handful of pumpkin seeds *or* a muesli made from oats, fresh hazelnuts, sunflower, pumpkin and sesame seeds and raisins with natural yoghurt and some apple juice.

- **Lunch:** A baked potato with tuna fish, tomato, celery and spring onion, with olive oil and lemon juice *or* a big rice salad with many types of fresh vegetables, cottage cheese, pumpkin seeds, olive oil, lemon juice and freshly ground black pepper.

- **Dinner:** Grilled fresh fish, chicken or lean meat or a vegetarian alternative made from beans, lentils or soya. Serve with a large helping of freshly steamed or lightly stir-fried vegetables. You can also 'steam-fry' vegetables by using just the tiniest drop of oil and adding a couple of tablespoons of water, to, in effect, steam them.

- **Snacks:** Fresh fruit, raw nuts and seeds (e.g. almonds, hazelnuts, Brazils, pumpkin and sunflower seeds); raw vegetables (e.g. carrots, broccoli, celery) with hoummous.

- **Drinks:** At least six glasses of water, herbal and fruit teas (beware of artificially flavoured or sweetened ones), fresh fruit and vegetable juices, occasional 'smoothies' – freshly made with fruits/fruit juices and yoghurt or soya milk.

THE REAL DANGERS OF SUGAR

We are all aware that sugar is not good for us – whether because it is 'fattening' or because it rots our teeth. But actually, the dangers of excess sugar intake go far deeper than that. Like oxidants, which are a major cause of ageing and degenerative disease, excess sugar in the blood is also very damaging. In a process called glycosylation, sugar (glucose) in the blood attaches itself to proteins until they can no longer function properly. All the cells in our bodies – including hormones, enzymes, immune cells, carriers for nutrients and other substances such as cholesterol and oxygen – are partly made of protein. If the protein is coated with glucose, it cannot get to its destination or do its job.

People with diabetes provide a clear illustration of the effects of excessive glycosylation. Because of a lack of insulin (which gets glucose into cells), diabetics have elevated blood sugar levels, which need to be controlled. They are particularly prone to hardening of the arteries, loss of nerve function, and eye and kidney disease, much of which is due to glycosylation. Although these are extreme effects in people with the serious condition, diabetes, they illustrate the damage caused by generally having too much glucose in your blood. The effects of this can be similar, on a lesser scale: a more subtle ageing, or impeding of the way cells work and repair themselves.

Such damage by excess glucose can have a significant effect on your skin. Collagen forms an integral part of the skin (see Chapter 2). Indeed it makes up around 40 per cent of the body's proteins, so if it is damaged in any way – by glycosylation or oxidation – the skin becomes saggy and wrinkled. Such changes also affect the efficiency with which skin cells are nourished, supplied with oxygen and unburdened of their waste products, which is bound to have an effect on the way they work and look. Another, less well understood way in which sugar affects skin is in the case of acne – people with acne have been shown to process sugar poorly. (For more on this, see Chapter 11.)

There are countless more reasons why sugar is a big no-no – not only sugar per se, but also refined carbohydrates such as white flour and many breakfast cereals which are converted into glucose during digestion. When any of these are consumed in excess of our energy needs, they are converted in the body into fats. You will see in the next chapter that it is only certain fats which contribute to the good health of our bodies and our skin, not those made from sugars. These fats can decrease the oxygen supply to cells, particularly those on the surface – i.e. skin and peripheries. To make matters worse, sugar prevents the release of the important fat, linoleic acid, from storage in the body, in effect creating a deficiency (see Chapter 10).

Sugars also slow down our immune response, which means we are less able to fight off infection. When we eat sugars and refined carbohydrates, they do not come naturally 'packaged' with the nutrients our bodies need to process them. This means they call on our reserves, depleting nutrients which could be used for more crucial purposes. For instance, sugar interferes with the way the body uses vitamin C, which is needed for the formation of collagen and elastin as well as for enhancing our immunity. What's more, sugar and refined foods create ideal conditions in the digestive tract for feeding yeasts and other unwanted organisms, as well as making digestion sluggish, which ultimately affects all parts of the body including the skin (see Chapter 7).

CHAPTER 23

WATER – NATURE'S MOISTURISER

Water is vital. All life on earth depends on it. Humans developed from creatures who lived in water. It is the most plentiful substance in our bodies – composing over 60 per cent of our body weight. Here are a few more surprising facts about water:

- The major ingredient in our blood, cells, muscles and bones is water.

- A person who weighs 65 kilos contains about 40 litres of water.

- Water is the key substance in most of the routine events that take place in the body.

- We need to take in about 2 litres of water daily for optimum body function – about half of this comes from our food (provided we eat plenty of fruit and vegetables) so the rest must come in the form of pure water.

CELL SUPPORT

Imagine a balloon filled with water – taut and firm to the touch. Let some of the water out and the balloon will shrink; the rubber may even become a little shrivelled. Deprive a cell of water and you will get a similar result – both its structure and the way it works will be diminished. The process of removing water – dehydration – leaves all our bodies' cells gasping for replenishment. And this applies particularly to skin cells which are exposed to the harsh elements of the outside world – including sun, cold, heating, air-conditioning and pollution. In normal body processes – through our skin, breathing out, via our kidneys and gut – we lose about 1.5 litres of water every day. (This does not even take into account the amount we lose during strenuous exercise or on a hot day.) So the logical answer to avoiding a deficit is to supply the cells with sufficient water and maintain the health of their membranes so that water does not escape unnecessarily.

RECOGNISING THIRST

Allowing yourself to become dehydrated seriously compromises your health – it damages your immunity, your cells' ability to regenerate and repair, your digestion, your energy production, your thought patterns and even your appetite control. Many of us have got used to ignoring our thirst mechanism – many of our clients say they don't drink water because they don't feel thirsty. Only when they start to increase their daily water intake do they realise what they have been depriving themselves of. Feeling hungry and tired between meals is sometimes actually due to your body's desire for water (i.e. thirst). By not giving it water you can end up eating too much or eating unhealthy snacks which contribute to the body's sugar or toxin load.

Small wonder, then, that ignoring your need for water affects every aspect of your body, not least your skin. Without an adequate supply of water, your cells cannot rebuild your body, nor can they clear waste products which stack up in the cells and your blood. This turns into a vicious cycle whereby the cells cannot receive enough oxygen or nutrients to work or cleanse properly. Deep in your skin, water is a crucial component, providing the basis of a healthy, soft and youthful complexion. Although very little water is actually stored in the outermost layers of your skin, this moisture is also important and is constantly being removed by outside elements.

Ironically, drinking more water often helps overcome water retention. Various factors can encourage water retention (see Chapter 21). These include kidney problems, food intolerance and eating too much sugar, but another is not drinking enough water. If you are not supplying your body with adequate water, it will make every effort to cling on to what it does have. Other drinks will not do, only pure water counts. Coffee and tea contain natural chemicals, including caffeine, which interfere with energy production, digestion, detoxification and much more. If you have herbal teas, make sure they are pure leaves or flowers of the plant (such as camomile or dandelion) and not flavoured tea which contains additives.

WATER PURITY

Having said this, the quality of the water you drink is also crucial – if it is contaminated with chemicals or metals (such as lead) it will pollute your body and interfere with all of its processes. Unfortunately, the vast majority of water supplies are contaminated and should be avoided. Instead, you should drink mineral water if you can afford it. Alternatively, use a good-quality water filter and change the filter regularly. Many companies now deliver mineral water or pure water in large 20-litre bottles, which can be an economical way of getting good-quality water for drinking and cooking. (see Useful Addresses or your local *Yellow Pages* for suppliers.)

....

CHAPTER 24

DETOXIFYING YOUR SKIN

Throughout the centuries, health experts have extolled the value of 'spring-cleaning' the body. In much the same way as you need a holiday from work, your body needs a break from its daily burden of toxins. One of the traditional methods of purifying the body is fasting. And the fact that many people say they feel so much more vital after fasting confirms the fact that making energy is as much a result of improving the body's ability to detoxify as it is about eating the right foods.

However, not everybody feels better from fasting and not always right away. A common occurrence is the so-called 'healing crisis' when a person feels worse for a few days and then feels better. The problem is that some of these people may be experiencing a real crisis, rather than a healing crisis. Once the body starts to liberate and eliminate toxic material, if the liver isn't up to the job, symptoms of intoxication can result. Hence, modern-day detox regimes tend to use modified fasts, in which the person is given a low-toxin diet, plus plenty of the key nutrients needed to speed up the body's ability to detoxify. Doing this once a year, for a couple of weeks, can make a major difference to your energy levels.

A more focused approach would involve consulting a clinical nutritionist (see Useful Addresses) and having a comprehensive detoxification profile test. On the basis of this, they will devise a specific diet and supplement programme to restore your detoxification potential to optimal levels. I have seen many long-term sufferers of skin problems such as acne (as well as other conditions such as chronic fatigue syndrome) completely recover within weeks of implementing a nutritional programme specifically designed to improve their detoxification potential.

The first step towards detoxifying the body is to remove or lessen the toxic load. Ideally we should minimise our toxic load all the time, but making a special effort for two weeks can be very cleansing and rejuvenating. Some foods contain and generate toxins, while others are very detoxifying. Most, however, have good factors and bad factors. Eating organic produce as far as possible also means that you are cutting down on the amount of toxins you are exposed to.

THE DETOX YOUR SKIN DIET

Beneficial foods

Foods that are definitely good for detoxification:

Fruit   The fruits with the highest detox potential include fresh apricots, all types of berries, cantaloupe melon, citrus fruits, kiwi, papaya, peaches, mango, melons, red grapes. Go easy on bananas (one a day only). Dried fruit is best avoided during these two weeks.

Vegetables   All are great but especially good ones include artichokes, peppers, beetroot, Brussels sprouts, broccoli, red cabbage, carrots, cauliflower, cucumber, kale, pumpkin, spinach, sweet potato, tomato and watercress. White potatoes and avocado should be eaten in moderation. Also excellent are sprouted beans and seeds. Try alfalfa, sprouted mung beans, chickpeas, lentils, aduki beans and sprouted sunflower seeds. These are available to buy, ready-sprouted, in most healthfood shops and some supermarkets and green grocers.

These foods (preferably organic) should make up the bulk of your two-week detox diet.

Limit

Foods that are generally good for you, but may contain low levels of toxins. They should make up no more than a third of your two-week diet.

Grains   Brown rice, corn, millet and quinoa.

Fish   Salmon, mackerel, sardines and tuna.

Meat   Organic skinless chicken, turkey and wild game.

Oils   Use extra-virgin olive oil for cooking in place of butter, and cold-pressed seed oils for dressing. Organic, cold-pressed flax oil is the best in this respect.

Nuts and seeds   A large handful a day of raw, unsalted nuts and seeds should be included in your diet. Try grinding them up and sprinkling them over a fruit salad. Include almonds, brazils, hazelnuts, pecans, pumpkin seeds, sunflower seeds, sesame seeds and flax seeds.

Avoid

The following foods, while normally OK in moderation, are best avoided during the two weeks because they are either hard to digest, mildly irritate the gut or are hard to detoxify.

Gluten grains   Barley, oats, rye and wheat (including spelt and kamut).

Meat and dairy produce   Milk and all dairy products, eggs and organic red meat.

Baddies

Foods that should be avoided at all times.

Red meat   Beef, pork and lamb.

Refined foods   White bread/pasta/rice.

Sugar   And any foods containing it.

Salt   And any foods containing it.

Hydrogenated or partially hydrogenated fat   Often used to make margarines.

Alcohol, tea, coffee and all soft drinks   including cola drinks and squash.

Other toxins   Also avoid as much as possible fried foods, pesticides, exhaust fumes and medications – most contain harmful substances that require detoxification.

Detox drinks

Needless to say, during these two weeks alcohol is out, as it is a major burden on the body. So too are any sources of 'methylxanthines', a family of chemicals that includes caffeine, tannin, theobromine and theophylline. This means no chocolate, coffee, tea or peppermint tea. Alternatives are shown below:

Fruit juice   Always dilute with an equal quantity of water.

Herbal teas   There is now a huge variety to choose from. Sample a few until you find one you like best.

Rooibosch tea   Caffeine-free and tastes very similar to 'normal' tea.

Dandelion coffee   Can be drunk as a coffee replacement whilst you are on your two-week detox diet. Once it is complete try Caro, Barleycup and Teechino.

Fruit or vegetable juice cocktails   Try a Virgin Mary or a watermelon juice or carrot and ginger juice.

Pure water   This is the best drink of all, so have lots of it. Drink 2 litres of purified, distilled, filtered or bottled water a day. This may seem like an awful lot to you. However, water puts no burden on your body and helps to dilute toxins as they are eliminated.

DETOX SUPPLEMENTS

Supplementing the nutrients that help your body to detoxify is a great way to speed up the benefits of this rejuvenating diet. The nutrients you need to support the first stage (Phase 1) of detoxification are vitamins B2, B3, B6, B12, folic acid, glutathione, branched chain amino acids, flavonoids and phospholipids, plus a good supply of antioxidant nutrients to disarm dangerous intermediary oxidants created during this phase.

Phase 2 of detoxification can be stimulated back into action by a specific list of nutrients including the amino acids glycine, taurine, glutamine and arginine. Cysteine, N-acetyl cysteine and methionine are also precursors for these nutrients (i.e. the body can convert these into the others).

You can help support detoxification by supplementing your detox diet with the following, all taken twice a day:

- multivitamin and mineral.

- antioxidant – choose a broad-spectrum supplement which contains a number of antioxidants such as vitamins A (beta carotene), C, E, glutathione, lipoic acid, selenium, zinc.

- vitamin C – 1000mg.

- milk thistle – 100mg.

• MSM – 1000mg.

(See Useful Addresses for suppliers.)

If you suspect that your skin problem may be connected with detoxification follow this regime for two weeks and see how you feel. Alternatively, you may prefer to consult a clinical nutritionist (see Useful Addresses), who will give you a comprehensive detoxification profile test. On the basis of this, he or she will devise a specific diet and supplement programme designed to restore optimal detoxification potential.

CHAPTER 25

LOW-REACTION DIETS

As you will have seen throughout this book, many skin problems can be caused by sensitivity to certain foods. This is not an absolute allergy as such, but a more subtle reaction, usually to a food that is eaten regularly such as wheat (found in bread, most cereals, pasta, pizza, biscuits, muffins and cakes) or dairy products such as milk or cheese.

Even more subtle are reactions to several foods which are usually linked to an over-sensitivity of the digestive tract, often caused by poor digestion (see Chapter 7). If a food is not digested well, usually due to insufficient digestive enzymes, it is likely to trigger a reaction in the gut, increase the amount of large molecules entering the bloodstream, or provide food for undesirable organisms which then multiply. If abnormally large particles of food pass through the intestinal lining, this then triggers an immune reaction elsewhere in the body which can show up as a skin condition (such as eczema) or some other problem such as low energy. (For more on allergies, see Chapter 18.)

FOOD ADDICTION

Another interesting finding among people with food sensitivities is that they are often hooked on the very food they are reacting to. This can lead to bingeing on the foods that harm them most. Many such people describe these foods as leaving them feeling dopey or giving them a temporary energy or mood lift. It is not known exactly how this works, but it is believed that proteins in such foods may act in a similar way to the body's natural endorphins, which switch off pain and give a natural 'high'.

Scientists have made endorphin-like substances from the proteins in wheat, milk, barley and corn and shown that they bind to the body's endorphin receptor sites. If you suspect that this may be the case, think of the foods you feel you 'couldn't live without' and you may well find that they are the ones you are sensitive to. If you stop eating the suspect foods, you may feel a little worse for a few days before you feel better, rather like going 'cold turkey' when giving up an addiction.

While food sensitivities may not necessarily be the root cause of a skin problem, they could well be an exacerbating factor and are well worth investigating with the help of a nutritionist or other health practitioner. There are several reasons why you may develop sensitivities: for instance, lack of digestive enzymes, leaky gut, frequent intake of gut irritants (such as chemicals, coffee and alcohol), lowered immunity or an over-proliferation of 'bad' bacteria in the gut. (For more on digestion, see Chapter 7).

ELIMINATION DIETS

It is essential to deal with the root cause of the sensitivities by identifying the most likely culprits. This is the key to overcoming food sensitivities. There are some diets which can be used to detect which foods are triggering a reaction, principally based on eliminating suspect foods.

Mono-elimination diet

Any one suspected food or food group should be avoided for at least two weeks. Choose to avoid, one at a time, from:

- Wheat products – bread, most cereals, pasta, pizza, biscuits, muffins, cakes, pastries and pies.

- Dairy products – anything made from or containing milk such as cheese, yoghurt or fromage frais.

- Eggs and anything containing eggs.

- Citrus fruits – oranges, tangerines, lemons, grapefruit and lime.

- Processed foods – anything containing preservatives, colouring and artificial flavouring.

While you are avoiding that particular food or food group notice any changes, or not, in your skin condition. After two weeks, reintroduce the food – have it two or three times a day for a few days to see if it triggers any reaction. If you do react when reintroducing it, go back to avoiding it. Otherwise, have it as you normally would. Once you've done this with one food, go on to the next and do the same.

Multi-elimination diet

In this diet, the most commonly allergy-provoking foods are eliminated from the diet, and any others that you know you are sensitive to, plus any that you eat almost daily. Those which should definitely be avoided are the ones listed under the mono-elimination diet, above. We very much recommend that you follow this diet under the guidance of an experienced health professional. With children, it is absolutely essential to have the guidance of an experienced practitioner to ensure that they are getting the full range of required nutrients.

Foods to include in the diet are:

- All vegetables (except potatoes, tomatoes and sweetcorn which are on the 'suspect' list).

- Fruits (pears, papaya and bananas are particularly unlikely to cause reactions)

- Rice, millet, buckwheat and quinoa (grains available in most healthfood stores).

- Oats, rye and barley (although some people are sensitive to the gluten they contain).

- Fresh, unprocessed, unsmoked meats and fish.

- Beans and lentils (although some people are sensitive to soya).

After four weeks of avoiding all these foods, each food is rein-troduced one by one, with a five-day gap before introducing the next one. This way it is clear which foods are producing symptoms or not. It may be worth drawing up a chart when you start reintroducing the foods – noting what you started eating, when and if you had any skin (or other) reactions.

If a food does trigger a reaction when it is reintroduced, it should be avoided for at least another six months, after which time you can retest by eating it again. During that avoidance time, you should work to improve your digestive and immune systems in order to minimise your chances of being sensitive to such foods.

CHAPTER 26

....

SUPPLEMENTS FOR CLEAR SKIN

In addition to following the Clear Skin diet in Chapter 22, it is definitely worth taking some supplementary nutrients. Your ideal intake will depend on your individual needs, your lifestyle, your diet and the environment in which you live. Remember, though, that supplements are just that – an addition to a good diet and healthy lifestyle, not a replacement for one.

For a personal dietary and supplement programme, tailored to your particular needs, it is best to consult a qualified nutritionist (see Useful Addresses). There are, however, some basic supplements for good health and great skin which can benefit everyone:

• A good multivitamin and mineral.

• Vitamin C (with bioflavonoids).

• An antioxidant blend (containing at least vitamins A, C, E, zinc, selenium and perhaps lipoic acid, glutathione, cysteine, lycopene, extracts of green tea, grape seed, pine bark or bilberry).

• An essential fatty acid supplement (perhaps linseed, fish or evening primrose oil or an oil blend).

• MSM (see below).

Individual brands will vary in exact content, so take them as directed on the bottle. Your nutritionist can advise you if you are in doubt. If you have a particular skin condition, taking extra doses of particular nutrients or other substances such as herbs can be very helpful – guidelines for these are given in each of the relevant chapters.

SULPHUR – THE MISSING NUTRIENT?

It is referred to in the Bible as brimstone and it is the fourth most abundant mineral in the body, but sulphur is often forgotten as a crucial element in health, including that of our skin and nails. This vital mineral is a constituent of keratin and collagen – substances in skin, nails and hair – so it's no surprise that they improve when people take supplements in the form of MSM (methyl sulfonyl methane).

So, rather than taking collagen, or using expensive creams that contain it, you're better off supplying your body with the raw materials it needs to make collagen such as MSM (along with vitamin C). Sulphur is needed for new cell formation (your skin is constantly renewing itself), and for keeping the bonds between cells pliable. It's also a great detoxifier. MSM has been shown not only to enhance the beauty of skin, nails and hair but also to help skin healing (e.g. after burns or wounds), acne, allergies, arthritis and much more. Start by taking 1000mg three times a day.

CHOOSING SUPPLEMENTS

As with any product, the quality of supplements varies considerably. Other than recommending particular brands, we always suggest that people do not go for the cheapest brands. The chances are that corners will have been cut – such as using a less absorbable form of nutrients or poorer-quality binders and fillers. There are even certain brands of vitamin C which add orange colouring and a sweetener – not my idea of optimum nutrition. Many of the companies will declare that their products are free of sugar, gluten, yeast, etc. So if you want a particular supplement and are in doubt, either choose a brand which lists all the ingredients or ask the manufacturer to supply a full list.

TAKING SUPPLEMENTS

Research into the importance of nutrition for healthy skin concludes that taking oral supplements has many benefits over topical application: it feeds skin over the entire body in a bioactive form and feeds even the deeper layers of the skin.[1] For youthful skin the best strategy is to do both.

While some supplements require a specific regime, most vitamins and minerals should be taken with meals (i.e. not more than 15 minutes before or after). Take most supplements earlier in the day (i.e. with breakfast or lunch) and don't take B vitamins at night if you have difficulty sleeping. If you are taking more than one vitamin B complex or C tablet, spread them throughout the day. Because nutrients work very much in synergy, it's best not to take individual minerals or individual B vitamins unless you are also taking a multinutrient supplement. Even then, these individual supplements are best taken under the guidance of a health practitioner.

CHAPTER 27

EXTERNAL SKINCARE

Surface skincare is potentially a minefield, especially when you consider that it is only one element in the whole equation of having clear skin. You could have the most efficient skincare routine imaginable, with excellent-quality products, but if you have a poor diet, bad digestive function, impaired liver detoxification, excessive sun exposure, you smoke, and you have inherited various genetic dispositions, it's unlikely to make a great deal of difference.

Then there are the lucky people. My mother has used nothing but an economical cleanser and moisturiser on her face all her adult life and looks gorgeous at 58; my aunt has immaculate skin, and uses nothing but a high street brand moisturiser. Or perhaps it's not just luck. The importance of the lifestyle factors I've mentioned above cannot be over-estimated. Having said that, it is also extremely important to take care of your skin from the outside, especially in today's environment which exposes us to the harsh effects of pollution, air conditioning and central heating.

We won't be going into too much detail about skin routine, as that's not the role of nutritionists and would warrant a book in itself anyway. The single most important step you can take is to follow the Clear Skin diet described in Chapter 22. Apart from that, you need to:

- Determine what type of skin you have, perhaps with the help of a trained skincare specialist.

- Clean your skin every day.

- Use a moisturiser (even oily skin needs protection).

- Keep your skin protected from the sun.

- Exfoliate regularly to remove dead cells.

DAILY CLEANSING

Daily cleansing is always vital – even if you do not wear make-up – as dirt and oils can clog your pores, causing blackheads and spots. The right cleanser will leave your skin feeling fresh and clean but not tight and dry. Make sure your cleanser is acid balanced (i.e. to the same pH as the skin, which is acidic with a pH of around 5.5). Acidity and alkalinity are measured on a scale from 1–14 called the pH scale; 7 is neutral and the lower the number, the more acidic.

Soap itself is very alkaline and washes away the skin's natural oils which are essential. Even if you have oily skin, removing all the oils will simply stimulate your skin to produce more. And if you live in a hard water area, it will dry out your skin further.

Cleansers which are not water-soluble need harsh alcohol-based toners to remove them from the skin and are probably clogging your pores and/or stripping them of natural oils. Choose a cleanser which rinses off easily with water and leaves some of the skin's oils so that it does not feel tight so you should not need a toner.

MOISTURISING

It may seem strange but *everyone* needs to moisturise (even people with oily skin). This isn't to add moisture as such, but to help the skin retain moisture. A good moisturiser, suited to your skin type, will help your skin retain water and protect it from the damaging effects of pollution and the sun.

If you have oily skin, choose a moisturiser which is completely oil-free but rich in hydrating substances such as microsponges or propylene glycol (i.e. binding water to the skin).

For dry skin, a richer moisturiser – not necessarily 'oilier' – leaves the skin protected and adds oil and water to it. Technology these days is such that you do not need to have a thick, oily moisturiser to do this.

EXFOLIATING

The process of removing the build-up of dead skin cells and any stubborn dirt from your skin is centuries old – even the ancient Egyptians used oatmeal to decongest the skin for renewal. As we age, the renewal rate of our skin slows down, which leaves it thicker and duller-looking. Whether you have dry or oily skin, regular exfoliation helps prevent it looking flaky or spotty.

There are two main methods – one is physical exfoliation, with grainy substances that work on the surface. However, natural substances are used in many skin creams these days as alternatives to physical abrasives which are too harsh for most skins. For example, alpha hydroxy acids (AHAs) are extracted from sugar cane, milk, molasses, apples or wine, and beta hydroxy acids (BHAs) from wintergreen and fruits, papain from papaya and bromelain from pineapples. These acids act by breaking down the intercellular 'glue' that holds cells together.

Don't be alarmed by images of facial disintegration! If well-formulated they form an important part of any skin routine. They help to clear blocked pores and smooth away dead, dry skin. If you have sensitive skin, go for a milder product with no more than 8 per cent AHAs – any higher may sting, although a very slight, temporary stinging is not unusual anyway. Again, it's always a good idea to get advice from an expert in a salon.

FEEDING YOUR SKIN

While feeding your skin from the inside is key to keeping it looking good, scientists have found that taking extra antioxidants (and other nutrients) may not always increase levels in the skin because the body cleverly routes ingested nutrients to more survival-orientated organs. Antioxidants – both ingested and put on the skin – have been shown conclusively to help prevent and treat sunlight-induced ageing and other skin conditions.[2] This is where antioxidant creams come in – only they too are susceptible to oxidation (see Chapter 3) in the jar and once on your skin, so they need to be well stabilised in order not to cause oxidant damage themselves.

Other than selling such creams in capsules, tubes or pump containers to protect them from air and light damage, companies can use particularly stable forms of the vitamins and combinations so that the various antioxidants can protect one another. For example, tocopheryl acetate is the stabilised form of vitamin E; it counters oxidants in the skin and jar; blended with ascorbic acid (one form of vitamin C) it protects beta carotene and retinyl palmitate (forms of vitamin A); and the vitamin C in turn protects the vitamin E. In other words, they 'recycle' one another. Good products will contain careful formulations which protect the vitamins and make them more likely to penetrate deeper into your skin.

Choosing a multivitamin cream

- Don't buy one in a jar, as the daily exposure to air increases the chances of oxidation. Single application capsules are ideal, otherwise tubes or pump action bottles.

- Look for a stabilised product. For instance, putting vitamin C in a lipid (oil) base gives it some protection from oxidation.

- Some good products encapsulate the vitamins in minute, envelope-like structures within the cream to protect them.

- Check where on the ingredients list the vitamins are – if they are right at the bottom, they are unlikely to be concentrated enough to make much difference.

PROTECTING YOUR SKIN FROM THE SUN

That the sun damages your skin is not news. Chapters 3, 4 and 9 will have underlined the importance of protecting your skin from sun exposure – not just to minimise your risk of skin cancer but also to avoid rapid ageing.

There are two main ways in which sunscreens work – either by physically blocking out the rays or by chemically absorbing them, dissipating the UV energy as heat. Chemical sunscreens include benzophenone and octyl methoxycinnamate, while titanium dioxide and zinc oxide provide physical barriers, actually reflecting the rays. The main difference is that the physical ones tend to leave a whitish colour on the skin (or very white, pink or green if you choose the cricketer or snowboarder look) but they are generally better for sensitive skins. Using a cream that contains both will give better protection, as different chemicals work best in protecting from different ends of the spectrum of light.

The SPF (sun protection factor) of a cream refers only to its protection from UVB rays (the 'burning' ones), not the UVA (longer-term, 'ageing' rays) and gives you an idea of how much extra time you can spend in the sun without burning. So if you usually burn after 20 minutes, an SPF 20 would protect you for $20 \times 20 = 400$ minutes (6 hours 40 minutes). However, it's now generally agreed that you should use at least an SPF 20 to protect yourself from skin damage, especially as you may not know exactly how long you take to burn or the effect of the environmental conditions (such as sun strength, altitude, etc).

Newer chemicals such as Parsol 1789 (chemical name: avobenzone) provide good protection from UVA rays. Better sunscreens also contain antioxidants, which protect the skin by mopping up oxidants as well as improving immune defences. Environ's RAD is my favourite (See Useful Addresses).

Make sure you use enough sunscreen and in good time – rubbing in a tiny amount half an hour after you've been out in the sun and have a sweaty sheen over your skin is going to make the cream more or less redundant. But remember, also, that the beach is not the only place you are exposed to the sun – just walking around on a sunny day puts you at risk of sun damage. And it's never too late to protect yourself. Even if you feel you could not do yourself any more harm than you have already done over the years, damage is cumulative so any protection is worthwhile.

If you *do* overdo it in the sun and get burnt, smother yourself in aloe vera gel or calamine lotion, and later use a good moisturiser. It's really too late for much skin rescue to be done – but if you are taking a good antioxidant supplement, you are at least doing some good from the inside.

As with any products, not all sunscreens are equally good. Research has shown that chemicals found in some sun creams may actually pass on excess energy from the sun's rays into the skin, where it damages DNA. These chemicals are Padimate-O, PABA-O or Escalol 507, says Dr John Knowland from Oxford University. The research was done in test-tubes, so it has yet to be discovered whether the same effect takes place in humans.[3] Norwegian scientists have recently shown a common sunscreen ingredient, octyl methoxycinnamate, to be harmful to the skin especially when it is exposed to UV rays.

Fake tans

You'll have realised by now that there really is no best way to tan. The best you can do is have no tan at all – unless you fake it. Thank goodness the days are long gone when a fake tan meant days of embarrassment afterwards because of ridiculous-looking apricot streaks giving away your secret. The discovery of dihydroxyacetone which really does turn brown on skin has revolutionised fake-tan products. There does not seem to be much difference between the products that contain this ingredient, so your choice should be based on your budget and the texture of the cream. Streaking can occur, however, if you have not exfoliated your skin well, as layers of dead skin will stain darker. So, exfoliate, spread the cream smoothly and evenly and remember to wash your hands well if you want to avoid tanned palms.

SKIN TREATMENTS

You can make your own face masks and cosmetics with various ingredients. One of the most effective and simple products is green clay (see Useful Addresses). Blending the clay with some water to form a paste and applying it to skin can draw out toxins and dirt, especially in the case of acne but also as a regular skin detoxifier; it also helps reduce inflammation and irritation. Leave it to dry on the skin (wash it off immediately if the skin feels sore) and rinse it off well. Mixing it with olive oil makes it more moisturising. Some people even advocate mixing the clay in a glass of water and drinking it (not the thicker sediment) to clean the digestive tract and draw out toxins.

Brushing your skin with a natural bristle brush is great not only for sloughing off dead cells but also for stimulating your lymph system and blood circulation which enhances the elimination of toxins as well as the delivery of oxygen and nutrients to cells. (See Chapter 17 for more on this.)

HARMFUL INGREDIENTS IN SKINCARE PRODUCTS

Certain ingredients are big no-nos in skin creams, while others are particularly aggravating for sensitive skin.

Ingredient	Used for	Reasons to avoid
Mineral oil – a petroleum by-product	A moisturiser; makes product feel 'silky'; adheres to skin surface	Leaves greasy after-feel; sits on surface; may trigger acne
Lanolin – derived from sheep wool or synthetic	A wax used as a moisturiser	May trigger acne or allergies; may contain carcinogens
Isopropyl myristate – derived from fatty alcohol	Makes product feel 'silky'; gives creams 'separability'	May trigger acne; penetrates and blocks hair follicles; causes blackheads
PABA – para aminobenzoic acid, a B vitamin	A sunscreening agent	Can trigger dermatitis in sensitive skin
SD alcohol – specially denatured alcohol	Astringent; antiseptic; makes fats soluble	Drying; irritating; dehydrates skin by removing moisture and sebum
Artificial fragrance	Disguising odours; 'signaturing' products	Can trigger allergies; can make skin more light-sensitive sensitive
D and C red dyes – coal tar derivatives	Colours product	Can trigger acne
Formaldehyde	Preservative (banned in Sweden and Japan)	Irritates skin; possibly carcinogenic
Urocanic acid – derived from animal or vegetable oils	Makes product spread better; often used in sunscreens	Can irritate skin; possibly carcinogenic
Phenol – carbolic acid	Antiseptic; often used in shaving creams	Can cause hives, stinging and rashes

Reprinted with kind permission of the International Dermal Institute, developers of Dermalogica skincare products

REFERENCES

Part 1

1 Kligman, A.M. et al., 'The anatomy and pathogenesis of wrinkles', *Brit J Dermatology* vol 113, pp 37–42 (1985).

2 Montagna, W. and Carlisle, K., 'Structural changes in aging human skin', *J Invest Dermatology* vol 73, p 47 (1979).

3 Schallreuter, K. and Wood, J., 'Free radical reduction in the human epidermis', *Free Rad Biol Med*, vol 6, pp 519–32 (1989).

4 Harley, C.B. et al., 'Telomeres shorten during aging of human fibroblasts', *Nature*, vol 345, pp 458–60, (1990).

5 Kedziora, J. and Bartosz, G., 'Downs syndrome: a pathology involving the lack of balance of reactive oxygen', *Free Radic Biol Med*, vol 4(5), pp 317–30 (1988).

6 Boyd, A.S. et al., 'Cigarette smoking-associated elastotic changes in the skin', *J Am Acad Dermatol*, vol 41(1), pp 23–6 (1999).

7 Tur, E. et al., 'Chronic and acute effects of cigarette smoking on skin blood flow', *Angiology*, vol 43(4), pp 328–35 (1992).

8 Thiele, J.J. et al., '*In vivo* exposure to ozone depletes vitamins C and E and induces lipid peroxidation in epidermal layers of murine skin', *Free Rad Biol Med*, vol 23, pp 385–91 (1997).

9 Fuchs, J. et al., 'Impairment of enzymic and nonenzymic antioxidants in skin by UVB radiation', *J Invest Dermatol*, vol 93, pp 769–73 (1989).

10 Eberlein-Konig, B. et al., 'Protective effect against sunburn of combined systemic ascorbic acid and d-alpha tocopherol', *J Am*

Acad Dermatol, vol 38, pp 45–8 (1998).
11 Fuchs, *op. cit.*

Part 2

1 Eberlien-Konig, B. et al., 'Protective effect against sunburn of combined systemic ascorbic acid (vitamin C) and d-alpha-tocopherol (vitamin E)', *J Am Acad Dermatol*, vol. 38, pp 45–8 (1998).
2 Potokar, M. et al., 'Effectiveness of vitamin E protecting against UV light – comparative testing of the natural tocopherols on the skin of the hairless mouse', *Fat Sci Technol*, vol 92, pp 406–10 (1994).
3 Shindo, Y. et al., 'Dose-response effects of acute ultraviolet irradiation of antioxidants and molecular markers of oxidation in murine epidermis and dermis', *J Invest Dermatol*, vol 102, pp 470–75 (1994).
4 Potapenko, A. et al., 'PUVA-induced erythema and changes in mechanoelectrical properties of skin. Inhibition by tocopherols', *Arch Dermatol Res*, vol 276, pp 12–16 (1984).
5 Roshchupkin, D. et al., 'Inhibition of ultraviolet light-induced erythema by antioxidants' *Arch Dermatol Res*, vol 266, pp 91–4 (1979).
6 Gollnick, H. et al., 'Systemic beta carotene plus topical UV sunscreen are an optimal protection against harmful effects of natural UV sunlight: results of the Berlin-Eilath Study', *Eur J Dermatol*, vol 6, pp 200–205 (1996).
7 Emonet-Piccardi N. et al., 'Protective effects of antioxidants against UVA-induced DNA damage in human skin fibroblasts in culture', *Free Radic Res* vol 29(4), pp 307–13 (1998).
8 See Wright, S., 'Essential Fatty Acids in Clinical Dermatology', *J Nutr Med*, vol 1, pp 301–13 (1990).

Part 3

1 Takayasu, S. et al., 'Activity of testosterone 5-alpha-reductase in various tissues of human skin', *J Invest Dermatol*, vol 74, pp 187–91 (1980).
Sansone, G. and Reisner, R., 'Different rates of conversion of

testosterone to dihydrotestosterone in acne and normal human skin: a possible pathogenic factor in acne', *J Invest Dermatol*, vol 56, pp 366–72 (1971).

2 Cohen, J. and Cohen, A., 'Pustular acne staphyloderma and its treatment with tolbutamide', *Can Med Assoc J*, vol 80, pp. 629–33 (1959).

3 Abdel, K. et al., 'Glucose tolerance in blood and skin of patients with acne', *Int J Derm*, vol 22, pp 139–49 (1977).

4 Juhlin, L. and Michaelsson, G., 'Fibrin microclot formation in patients with acne'. *Acta Derm Venereol* vol 63(6), pp 538–40 (1983).

5 Bassett, I.B. et al., 'A comparative study of tea tree oil versus benzoyl peroxide in the treatment of acne', *Med J Aust*, vol 153, pp 455–8 (1990).

6 Sibenge, S. and Gawkrodger D., 'Rosacea: a study of clinical patterns, blood flow and the role of Demodex folliculorum', *J Am Acad Dermatol*, vol 26(4), pp 590–3 (1992).

7 Burton, J.L. et al., 'The sebum excretion rate in rosacea', *Br J Dermatol*, vol 92(5), pp 541–3 (1975).

8 Ryle, J. and Barber, H., 'Gastric analysis in acne rosacea', *Lancet*, vol 2, pp 1195–6 (1920).

9 Barba, A. et al., 'Pancreatic exocrine function in rosacea', *Dermatologica*, vol 165, pp 601–6 (1982).

10 Tulipan, L. 'Acne rosacea: a vitamin B complex deficiency', *NY State J Med*, vol 29, pp 1063–4 (1929).

11 Erbagci, Z. and Osgoztasi, O., 'The significance of Demodex follicularum density in rosacea', *Int J Dermatol*, vol 37(6), pp 421–5 (1998).

Sibenge, S. and Gawkrodger D., op. cit.

12 Roihu, T. and Kariniemi, A.L., 'Demodex mites in acne rosacea', *J Cutan Pathol*, vol 25(10), pp 550–2 (1998).

13 Johnson, L. and Eckardt, R., 'Rosacea, keratitis and conditions with vascularization of the cornea treated with riboflavin', *Arch Opth*, vol 23, p 899 (1940).

14 Studzinski, G.P. and Moore, D.C., 'Sunlight – can it prevent as well as cause cancer?', *Cancer Res*, vol 55(18), pp 1014–22 (1995).

15 Pathak, M., 'Activation of the melanocyte system by ultra-

violet radiation and cell transformation', *Ann NY Acad Sci*, vol 453, pp 328–39 (1985).

16 'Food, Nutrition and the Prevention of Cancer', World Cancer Research Fund, American Institute for Cancer Research (1997).

17 Weber, G., 'Cytoendocrinological findings in the pituitary glands of patients with psoriasis', *Acta Endocrinol (Cophenh)*, vol 119(4), pp 501–5 (1988).

18 Prystowsky, J.H. et al., 'Update on nutrition and psoriasis', *Int J Dermatol*, vol 32(8), pp 582–6 (1993).

19 Davies, S. and Stewart, A., *Nutritional Medicine*, Pan Books (1987).

20 Cant, A.I. et al., 'Effect of maternal dietary exclusion on breast-fed infants with eczema: two controlled studies', *Br Med J*, vol 293, pp 231–3 (1986).

21 Burks, A.W. et al., 'Peanut protein as a major cause of adverse food reaction in patients with atopic dermatitis', *Allergy Proceed*, vol 10, pp 265–9 (1989).

22 Lever, R. et al., 'Randomised controlled trial of advice on an egg exclusion diet in young children with atopic eczema and sensitivity to eggs', *Pediatr Allergy Immunol*, vol 9(1) (1998).

23 Majamaa, H. and Isolauri, E., 'Evaluation of the gut mucosal barrier: evidence for increased antigen transfer in children with atopic eczema', *J Allergy Clin Immunol*, vol 91, pp 668–79 (1996).

24 Savolainen, J. et al., 'Candida albicans and atopic dermatitis', *Clin Exp Allergy*, vol 23, pp 332–9 (1993).

25 Sakai, A. et al., 'Fatty acid compositions of plasma lipids in atopic dermatitis/asthma patients', *Arerugi*, vol 43(1), pp 37–43 (1994).

26 David, T.J., 'Serum levels of trace metals in children with atopic eczema', *Br J Dermatol*, vol 122, pp 485–9 (1990).

27 Amellal, M. et al., 'Inhibition of mast cell histamine release by flavonoids and bioflavonoids', *Planta Med*, vol 61, pp 16–20 (1985).

28 McNally, N.J. et al., 'Atopic eczema and domestic water hardness', *Lancet*, vol 352(9127), pp 527–31 (1998).

29 Rosenbaum, M. et al., 'An exploratory investigation of the

morphology and biochemistry of cellulite', *Plast Reconstr Surg*, vol 101(7), pp 1934–9 (1998).

30 Bourguignon, Di, 'Study of the action of titrated extract of Centella asiatica', *Gazette Med Fr*, vol 82, pp 4579 (1982).

31 Ormerod, A.D. et al., 'Penicillin in milk – its importance in urticaria', *Clin Allergy*, vol 17, pp 229–34 (1987).

32 Winkelman, R.K., 'Food sensitivity and urticaria or vasculitis', in Brostoff and Challacombe (eds.), *Food Allergy and Intolerance*, W.B. Saunders (1987).

33 Juhlin, L., 'Additives and chronic urticaria', *Ann Allergy*, vol 59, pp 119–23 (1987).

Zuberbier, T. et al., 'Pseudoallergen-free diet in the treatment of chronic urticaria', *ACTA Dermatologica Venerol (Stockh)*, vol 75, pp 484–7 (1995).

Part 4

1 Richelle, M. et al. 'Skin bioavailability of dietary vitamin E, carotenoids, polyphenols, vitamin C, zinc and selenium', *British Journal of Nutrition*, vol 9, pp 227–38 (2006).

2 Keller, K.L. and Fenske, N.A., 'Uses of vitamins A, C and E and related compounds in dermatology: a review', *J Am Acad Dermatol*, vol 39, pp 611–25 (1998).

3 Knowland, J. and McHugh, P.J., 'Characterisation of DNA damage inflicted by free radicals from a mutagenic sunscreen ingredient and its location using an in vitro genetic reversion assay', *Photochem Photobiol*, vol 66(2), pp 267–81 (1997).

RECOMMENDED READING

General

The New Ageless Ageing, Leslie Kenton, Vermilion (1995)
Perfect Skin, Amanda Cochrane, Piatkus (2000)
Optimum Wellness, Ralph Golan, Ballantine Books, New York (1995)
The Optimum Nutrition Cookbook, Patrick Holford and Judy Ridgway, Piatkus (1999)
Skin Secrets, Professor Nicholas Lowe, MD, and Polly Sellar, Collins & Brown (1999)
Boost Your Immune System, Patrick Holford and Jennifer Meek, Piatkus (1998)
Jane Scrivner's Total Detox, Jane Scrivner, Piatkus (2000)

Part 2

Gut Reaction, Gudrun Jonsson, Vermilion (1999)
The 20-Day Rejuvenation Diet Programme, Jeffrey Bland, PhD, Keats Publishing (1997)
Improve Your Digestion, Patrick Holford, Piatkus (1999)
Liver Detox Plan, Xandria Williams, Vermilion (1998)
Say No to Cancer, Patrick Holford, Piatkus (1999)
Fats that Heal Fats that Kill, Udo Erasmus, Alive Books (1996)

Part 3

Daylight Robbery, Dr Damien Downing, Arrow Books (1988)
The 30-Day Fatburner Diet, Patrick Holford, Piatkus (1999)
Beat Stress and Fatigue, Patrick Holford, Piatkus (1999)

Part 4

Supplements for Superhealth, Patrick Holford, Piatkus (1999)
The MSM Miracle, Earl Mindell, Keats Publishing (1997)

Useful Addresses

Organisations

National Eczema Society
163 Eversholt Street, London NW1 1BU
Tel: 0800 089 1122 (Helpline)
Website: www.eczema.org

Acne Support Group
Howard House, The Runway, South Ruislip, Middlesex HA4 6SE
Tel: 020 8561 6868
Website: www.yourskin.co.uk
Email: asg@the-asg.demon.co.uk

Psoriasis Association
7 Milton Street, Northampton NN2 7JG
Tel: 08456 760076
Website: www.psoriasis-association.org.uk

Nutrition Consultation
For a personal referral by Patrick Holford to a nutritional therapist in your area, visit www.patrickholford.com and select 'advice' for an immediate online referral. This service gives details on whom to see in the UK as well as internationally. If there is no-one available nearby you can always do an online assessment – see below.

Nutrition Assessment Online
You can have your own personal health and nutrition assessment online using the 100% Health Programme. Visit www.patrickholford.com.

Institute for Optimum Nutrition (ION)

The Institute for Optimum Nutrition (ION) offers a three-year foundation degree course in nutritional therapy. There is a clinic, a list of nutrition practitioners across the UK, an information service and a quarterly journal – *Optimum Nutrition*. Contact ION at Avalon House, 72 Lower Mortlake Road, Richmond TW9 2JY

Tel: 020 8614 7800

Website: www.ion.ac.uk.

Food allergy and intolerance

YorkTest also sell a home test kit for food allergies that requires a pinprick blood sample. YorkTest laboratories will test you for sensitivity to all foods including gluten, gliadin, wheat and yeast. They send you a home test kit that enables you to take a pinprick of blood, so you don't have to go to your doctor. Call them for a clinically proven test kit for simple blood collection at home; laboratory analysis, results within ten days.

Tel: 0800 074 6185

Website: www.yorktest.com.

Psychocalisthenics

Psychocalisthenics is an excellent exercise system that takes less than twenty minutes a day, and develops strength, suppleness and stamina and generates vital energy. The best way to learn it is to do the Psychocalisthenics Training. See www.patrickholford.com/psychocalisthenics for details on these. Also available in the book *Master Level Exercise: Psychocalisthenics*, the *Psychocalisthenics* CD and DVD.

Salt alternatives

The average person gets far too much sodium because we eat too much salt (sodium chloride) and salted foods, and not enough potassium and magnesium, found in fruit and vegetables. The net result is water retention and weight gain, anxiety, insomnia, high blood pressure and muscle cramps. Not all salt, however, is bad for you. Solo Low Sodium Sea Salt contains 60 per cent less sodium and is high in the essential minerals magnesium and potassium. Their 200g reusable shaker is sold in the UK, Ireland, Spain, Netherlands, Singapore, Hong Kong, Japan, Bahrain, Saudi Arabia, United Arab Emirates, Jordan, Baltic States and United States of America.

Tel: +44 (0)845 130 4568 (International Helpline)

Website: www.soloseasalt.com

Skin-care Products
Environ products were developed by cosmetic surgeon Dr Des Fernandes to address the damaging effects of the environment on our skin. Formulated with scientifically proven active ingredients including Vitamin A and antioxidant vitamins C, E and beta-carotene, which are used in progressively higher concentrations, Environ will maintain a normal healthy skin, especially when there are signs of ageing, pigmentation, problem skin and scarring. Their core vitamin A range is called AVST, which includes facial creams and Vitamin ACE body oil. They also provide C-Boost, a vitamin C rich skin cream and an excellent sun screen called RAD.

Environ products are available from Totally Nourish:
Tel: 0800 085 7749 (freephone)
Website: www.totallynourish.com

For international Environ enquiries call +2721 683 1034, or go to factory@environ.co.za. Environ products are also available from skin care therapists (see below).

Skincare Therapists
The International Institute for Anti-Ageing (iiaa) provides professional training and information to skincare therapists about the latest anti-ageing treatments and products. These well-informed therapists provide iiaa recommended, science-backed skincare (Environ) and nutritional products which are formulated to maintain and support healthy skin. They use their knowledge and experience to help you to address your skin concerns from both inside and out. To find your nearest iiaa trained therapist:
Tel: 020 8450 7997
Website: www.iiaa.eu

Water filters
There are many water filters on the market. One of the best is offered by the Fresh Water Filter Company who produce mains-attached water-filtering units. For details:
Tel: 0800 085 7749 (freephone in the UK)
Website: www.totallynourish.com

Supplement and Product Suppliers

Biocare produce a wide range of supplements including digestive and detoxification formulas, essential fat blends and MSM.
BioCare Ltd, Lakeside, 180 Lifford Lane, Kings Norton, Birmingham B30 3NU.
Tel: 0121 433 3727
Website: www.biocare.co.uk

Solgar produce a wide range of supplements which are widely available in healthfood shops and pharmacies.
Solgar Vitamins Ltd., Beggars Lane, Aldbury, Tring, Herts HP23 5PT
Tel: 01442 890355 for your nearest stockist
Website: www.solgar.co.uk

The Nutri Centre sells a very wide range of brands of supplements and creams. In addition to a large stock (which can be bought by mail order), they are very good at tracking down more obscure products.
The Nutri Centre, Unit 3, Kendal Court, Kendal Avenue, London W3 0RU
Tel: 0845 6026774
Fax: 020 8993 2188
Website: www.nutricentre.com

Neal's Yard Remedies sell herbs, essential oils and other natural cosmetics by mail order. They have shops throughout Britain.
Tel: 0161 831 7875 for mail order

Eco-co products sell eco-balls and environmental cleaning products.
The Barley Mow Centre, 10 Barley Mow Passage, Chiswick, W4 4PH
Tel: 0845 230 4200
Website: www.ecozone.co.uk

Supplements
Biocare's **Histazyme Plus** can be very helpful in counteracting skin reactions such as hives. **Digestpro** from the Patrick Holford Range contains both probiotics, plus digestive enzymes. The **Optimum Nutrition Pack** also from the Patrick Holford range contains multivitamins & minerals, plus vitamin C & zinc, and essential omega 3 and 6 fats. Vitamin C & Lysine tablets are also available from BioCare. **Super Lysine Plus** cream is made by Quantum and is available from The Nutri Centre.

INDEX

absorption 4
aciclovir 123
acne 69–76
acne conglobata 69
acne rosacea 77–81
acne vulgaris 69
addiction, food 151–2
additives 116–17
  food 100
adult acne 72–3
ageing 14, 20, 50, 51
air pollution 17
alcohol 88, 148
allergens 113
allergic reactions 113
allergies 113–14
  food 100–1
aloe vera 81
  gel 84, 133, 163
alpha hydroxy acids (AHA) 160
alpha-linolenic acid family *see* omega 3
androgens 25, 26
animal fats 95
anthocyanidins 53, 57–8
anti-allergy nutrients 119
antibiotics 39, 72, 115
antioxidant creams 161
antioxidants 15, 18, 22, 50–9, 155
  supplements 50, 53, 58–9
arginine 122, 123, 149
aspirin 115, 117
athlete's foot 125, 127
atopic eczema 98
avoidance diets 101
avoidance testing 118–19, 129

bacteria 38–9, 94, 99
Baker, S. 48
bathing, sea 93
beneficial bacteria 126
benzoyl peroxide 74
Berwick, M. 88
beta hydroxy acids (BHA) 160
beta-carotene 51, 53, 55
bifido bacteria 126

bioflavonoids 53, 111, 119, 123
biotin 103
biotransformation 46
blackheads 7, 69, 70
Bland, J. 44
blood clots 83
body temperature 4
borage oil 65
bowel toxins 71
bowels 71–2
breast cancer 87
breast-feeding 100, 127
bromelain 94
burns 85
burnt food 88

caffeine 148
calamine lotion 163
camomile 93
cancer 22
  risk 87
Candida albicans 40, 94, 101
capillaries 16–17
carbohydrates 38
carotene 8
cayenne pepper extract 93
cells
  exchange between 109
  membrane 16, 65
  replication 83
cellulite 106–12
cellulitis 106
chain amino acids 149
chemical sunscreens 162
chemicals 28, 115–16
chia oil 63
chia seeds 63
chicken pox 4
chromium 71
cleaning products 105
cleansers 75
cleansing 74, 159
clear skin diet 137–9
clogging substances 74
clove oil 133

coal tar preparations 92
cod liver oil 63
coenzyme Q10 (Co-Q10) 51, 56
coffee 144, 148
cold sores 4, 121–4
collagen 11–12, 57, 83, 140
colour, skin 7–8
conjugation 48
connective tissue 11, 107, 112
constipation 72, 109
corticosteroid creams 99
cotton clothing 105
cysteine 56–7, 149

D and C dyes 74
dairy products 72, 100, 129, 147
dandelion coffee 148
Davies, S. 100
dehydration 143
delta-6-desaturase enzyme 102
Demodex folliculorum 78, 80
dermatitis 98
  contact 98, 104
dermis 6–7
detoxification 43–9, 145–50
  tests 45–6, 145
detoxification capacity 44–6
  protection 49
DGLA (di-homo gamma linolenic acid) 64
DHA (docosahexaenoic acid) 62, 63, 64
DHT (dihydrotestosterone) 70
diabetes 140
diadzein 29
diet 95–7, 137–41
  acne 70–1
  acne rosacea 79
  avoidance 101
  cellulite 111
  clear skin 137–9
  eczema 100
  elimination 117, 152–4
  healing 84
  low reaction 151–4
  toxin-free 109
digestion 35–42, 151
digestive juices 38
digestive tract 36, 71–2, 116
  see also gut health; leaky gut syndrome
dimpling 107
dithranol 92

diuretics 129
DNA (deoxyribonucleic acid) 16, 22
drinks, detoxification 148
dust mites 105

E102 117
eco-balls 105
eczema 98–105
EFA *see* essential fatty acids
eggs 100, 101
elastin 12, 16
elimination 4
elimination diets 117, 152–4
ELISA (enzyme linked immuno sorbent assay) 118
emollients 92, 99
endo-toxins 43
endorphins 152
energy production 18
environmental oestrogens 27–8
enzymes 94
EPA (eicosapentaenoic acid) 62, 63, 64
epidermis 5–6
Escalol 507: 163
essential fats 60–6, 73, 96, 102, 103, 141
essential fatty acids (EFA) 60–6, 102, 131, 155
  deficiencies 63, 64, 65, 129
evening primrose oil 65
exercise 38, 110, 111, 112
exfoliating 160–1
exo-toxins 43

facial puffiness 128–30
fair skin 87
fake tans 163–4
fasting 145
fat 60, 109–10
fat chambers 107, 110
fats *see* essential fats
feeding, skin 161–2
fish 63, 96, 100, 102, 103, 147
fish oils 63, 96
flavonoids 104, 149
flax seed oil 63, 96
flax seeds 63
folic acid 96, 149
food 116, 146–8
  addiction 151–2
  additives 100
  allergies 100–1

burnt 88
  fresh 117, 126
  fried 88
  high-antioxidant 88
  processed 62, 111
  refined 148
  sensitivities 36, 151, 152
freckles 22
free oxidising radicals *see* oxidants
free radicals *see* oxidants
fresh food 117, 126
fried fats 96
fried food 88
fruit 146
fruit juice 148
fungal infections 125–7

gamma-linolenic acid (GLA) 63
garlic 126, 131, 133
gastrointestinal infections 36
gastrointestinal permeability 36
genistein 28
genital herpes 122
genital warts 133
glucose *see* sugar
glutamine 149
glutathione 48, 56–7, 149
glutathione lipoic acid 51
gluten 100
gluten grains 147
glycine 149
glycosylation 139–40
glycyrrhetinic acid 93, 104
Gotu kola 84–5, 112
grains 147
green clay 164
gut health 93–4, 101–2
  see also digestive tract; leaky gut
    syndrome

haemoglobin 8
harmful ingredients, skincare products
    165
healing 82–5
  crisis 145
hemp seeds 96
herbal teas 148
herbs 94–5, 129
Herpes virus 123
  simplex I 121
  simplex II 122

high-antioxidant foods 88
histamine 113
hives 113–19
homocysteine 48
hormones 25–7
hydrochloric acid (HCl) 78, 79, 80,
    132
hydrogenated fat 148
hydroxyproline 12

ideal weight 110
IgA (secretory immunoglobulin A) 36
immune response 141
immune system 36, 99, 123
impetigo 130–1
indigestion 38
inflammation 36, 82
insulin 71, 72
intestines *see* digestive tract
isoflavones 29
isopropyl myristate 74
isotretinoin (Roaccutane) 75

jock itch 125

keloid scars 83
keratin 6, 70
keratinocytes 21
Knowland, J. 163

lactic acid 38
Lactobacillus acidophilus 126
Langerhan cells 23
lanolin 74
lavender oil 127
leaky gut syndrome 36, 41, 101
lecithin granules 96
lemon balm 123
leukotrienes 117
licorice 104
linoleic acid 64, 102, 141
linoleic acid family *see* omega 6
linseed oil 102
linseeds 96
lip problems 131–2
lipase production 80
lipoic acid 58
liver 38, 43, 95
low reaction diets 151–4
lymph nodes 107
lymph vessels 8–10

lymphatic drainage massage 111
lymphatic system 107, 109
lysine 122, 123

magnesium 103, 129
meat 147, 148
melanin 7–8, 21
melanoma 87–8
menopause 26–7
menstrual cycle 122
methionine 149
methotrexate 93
methylxanthines 148
milk 72, 100
milk thistle 95
minerals 155
moisturisers 75
moisturising 159–60
moles 89
mono-elimination diet 152–3
mono-unsaturated fat 60
mouth, lines around 17
MSM (methyl sulfonyl methane) 156
Multi-elimination diet 153
multivitamin cream 161–2
multivitamins 155

N-acetyl-cysteine 56–7, 149
nails 31–2, 126
nappy rash 125
natural defences, against sun 21–2
nerves 4
nutrients 13, 111–12
    see also minerals; proteins; vitamins
nuts 147

octyl methoxycinnamate 163
oedema 117
oestrogen 25, 26, 27
    environmental 27–8
oils 147
omega 3: 60, 62–4, 102, 103
omega 6: 60, 64–5, 103
'orange peel' *see* cellulite
oregano 94
oregon grape 94
organs, priorities 10
oxidants 14–18, 88
    minimising exposure 16–18
    unavoidable 18
oxidation 14–18, 51, 53

oxidative damage 20
oxygen 15, 51
ozone 17, 19–20, 21

P-450 enzymes 46
PABA-O 163
Padimate-O 163
pancreatic lipase 78
paronychia 126
'PCB-free' 64
peanuts 100
penicillin 115
phospholipids 149
physical barriers, sunscreens 162
physiological weaknesses, eczema 99
phytates 28
phyto-oestrogens 28–9
plantar warts 133
pollution, air 17
polymorphic light eruption (PLE) 23
polyunsaturated fats 60
pores 74
potassium 129
prickly heat 114
priorities, organs 10
probiotics 39, 126
processed foods 62, 111
products, aggravate eczema 104
progesterone 25
Proprionibacterium acnes 70
prostaglandins 62–3, 64
protease 94
proteins 38, 96, 140
psoraisis 90–7
psoralens 93
puberty 25–6
pumpkin seed oil 96
pumpkin seeds 96
pycnogenol 53

quercetin 95, 104, 119
questionnaire, detoxification capacity
    44–5

rashes 4, 113–19
RAST (radioallergosorbent test) 118
raw vegetables 111
refined food 148
retinoids 93
rhinophyma 77
ringworm 125
Rooibosch tea 148

safflower oil 96
salicylic acid 93
salt 148
sarsparilla 94
saturated fat 60
scabs 83
scars 83
scurvy 12
sebaceous glands 7
seborrhoeic dermatitis 98
sebum 7, 69, 70, 78
seed oils 64–5
seeds 64, 96, 103, 147
selenium 51, 55, 56
self-confidence *see* self-image
self-image 4, 73, 77, 90
sensitivity
    to food 36, 151, 152
    to ultraviolet light 23
skin
    colour 7–8
    function 4–10
    living organ 3, 10
    structure 5–10
skin brushing 111, 164
skin cancer 86–9
skincare 4–5
    external 158–65
    products, harmful ingredients 165
skin mites 78, 80
skin prick test 118
skin treatments 164
smoking 16–17, 88
soap 159
soya 28
SPF (sun protection factor) 162
spot creams 74
spots 69, 70
staphyloccocus bacteria 130
Staphylococcus aureus 99
steroids 93
stomach acid *see* hydrochloric acid
stratum corneum 6, 22
strength 11–13
stress 36, 72–3, 78, 92, 105, 120, 121–2
stretch marks 11
sugar 71, 126, 131, 139–41, 148
sulphur 95, 156
sun 19–24
    minimising damage 23–4
    protection from 162–4

sun protection factor (SPF) 162
sunburn 20
sunflower oil 96
sunlight 86–7, 93
sunscreens 88, 162
suntans 21
supplements 95–7, 103–4, 155–7
    choosing 156–7
    detoxification 149
    taking 157
suppleness 11–13
sweat glands 8
sweating 8
Swedish bitters 94
synergy 53–4

tannin 148
tartrazine 117
taurine 149
tea 144, 148
tea tree oil 75, 84, 126, 131
teens 25–6
testing, allergies 118–19
testosterone 26, 27, 69–70, 73
theobromine 148
theophylline 148
thickness 22
thioctic acid 58
thirst 143–4
thrush 40, 125
Thuja oil 133
tinea pedis 125
tocopheryl acetate 161
toxic load 146
toxin-free diet 109
toxins 38, 43, 48–9, 94, 95, 111
'trans' fats 62
treatment
    acne 73–6
    acne rosacea 79–81
    allergies 119–20
    cellulite 110–12
    cold sores 122–4
    eczema 101–5
    fungal infections 126–7
    psoriasis 92–7
tretinoin (Retin–A) 74
tricolosan 75

ultraviolet C 20
ultraviolet light therapy 93, 99

ultraviolet rays *see* UV light
unidentified faecal organisms (UFO)
    39–40
urticaria *see* hives
UV light 19–21, 54–5
    UVA rays 20, 88–9
    UVB rays 20, 22, 89

vegetables 146
    raw 111
verrucae 133
vinegar 127
vitamin C cream 133
vitamin E oil 84
vitamins
    A 51, 53, 54–5, 73, 95, 103, 131
    B 78, 103, 131, 132, 157
    B2: 149
    B3: 103, 149
    B6: 73–4, 103, 149
    B12: 149
    C 12, 13, 22, 51, 53, 54–5, 95, 103,
        111, 119, 123, 131, 132, 141, 155
    D 86, 93
    E 22, 51, 53, 54–5, 103
vitiligo 132

warts 133–4
water 142–4, 149
    intake 12, 13
    purity 144
    retention 117, 128, 144
watermelons 55
weight control 110
wheat products 129
whiteheads 69
wound healing 82–4
wrinkles 12

xeno-oestrogens 27

yeasts 94
yellowish skin tone 4
yoghurt 126

zinc 51, 55, 56, 73, 95, 103, 123, 131, 132